# Relational Theory for Social Work Practice

*Relational Theory for Social Work Practice* introduces social workers to the burgeoning feminist scholarship on relational theories and the practical application of these theories with diverse populations. It emphasizes the practical application of the basic relational concepts in a readable and comprehensive way, developing an approach to practice that is useful for both male and female social workers and clients.

Relational theory argues that the fundamental feature of healthy human development is the ability to form connections through relationships. Within this perspective, growth is seen as occurring within relationships rather than apart from them. Relational theory from a feminist perspective brings together two disciplines that share the view that connection and affiliative needs are crucial to the development of self.

This work builds explicitly on the professional foundation of social work: mission, theory, practice skills, ethics, and values. Full case studies viewed through a feminist lens are integrated throughout the book. Helpful pedagogical features include a list of best practices for the social worker and a relational questionnaire. It will be of interest to students, researchers, and social work professionals.

**Sharon Freedberg** is an Associate Professor in the Social Work Department at Lehman College, City University of New York, USA.

# Relational Theory for Social Work Practice

## A Feminist Perspective

**Sharon Freedberg**

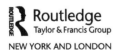

Routledge
Taylor & Francis Group

NEW YORK AND LONDON

First edition published 2009
by Routledge
270 Madison Ave, New York NY 10016

Simultaneously published in the UK
by Routledge
2 Park Square, Milton Park, Abingdon, Oxon, OX14 4RN

*Routledge is an imprint of the Taylor & Francis Group, an informa
business*

Transferred to Digital Printing 2010

© 2009 Taylor & Francis

Typeset in Sabon by
RefineCatch Limited, Bungay, Suffolk

*Library of Congress Cataloging in Publication Data*
Freedberg, Sharon, 1947–
Relational theory for social work : a new paradigm for practice /
Sharon Freedberg.
p. cm.
ISBN 978–0–7890–1263–0 — ISBN 978–0–7890–1264–7
1. Social case work.   I. Title.
HV43.F74 2008
361.3'201—dc22

                                                    2008008129


ISBN10: 0–7890–1263–4 (hbk)
ISBN10: 0–7890–1264–2 (pbk)
ISBN10: 0–203–88370–5 (ebk)

ISBN13: 978–0–7890–1263–0 (hbk)
ISBN13: 978–0–7890–1264–7 (pbk)
ISBN13: 978–0–203–88370–9 (ebk)

Dedicated to the memory of my mother and father,
who taught me the meaning of give and take

# Contents

# Preface

When existing theories are inadequate to explain anomalies of information in the real world, a crisis may emerge. According to Thomas Kuhn (1970), science does not develop by the accumulation of individual discoveries and inventions. Instead, the accretion of knowledge and scientific developments evolves into a new paradigm in which rules, laws, facts, and principles are structurally linked in a radically different way to explain existing phenomena. The goal of any new paradigm is to allow for the closest possible fit between empirical facts, changes in perceptions, history, and the nature of the social environment.

Since the rise of the feminist movement in the 1960s, a proliferation of feminist scholarship, along with changes in gender relations, have challenged women's realities and questioned the use of male-oriented empirical evidence and theory to explain female growth and behavior. Female writers have demonstrated that traditional psychological, cognitive, and social theories and forms of practice neglected or misunderstood many aspects of women's experience; in particular, gender-specific relational processes. In light of these developments, Kuhn's ideas took on heightened significance for me, helping me to recognize the need for a new and innovative paradigm for social work practice—one that stresses social work's relational elements.

Partially in response to this gap in theory and knowledge, I turned to the feminist-oriented relational-cultural perspective as a needed additive to the foundation for social work practice. Furthermore, my interest in writing a book on feminist relational-cultural theories and their relation to practice stems from my long-held belief that, while social work is a female-dominated profession, its hierarchy and knowledge base reflect the larger male-oriented society. My review of social work foundation texts reveals a predominance of traditional male-oriented theories of development that emphasize separation/individuation rather than highlighting the role that connection plays in adaptation and development.

Relational theory from a feminist perspective brings together writers who share the view that connection and affiliative needs are crucial to the development of self. Most importantly, relational theory posits that relationship is the cornerstone of human development and, therefore, any notion of autonomy and/or separation-individuation must be seen as occurring *within* relationship rather than *apart* from relationship. The social organization of roles in a patriarchal society mirrors power inequality between women and men and, hence, prevailing theories in institutionalized professions such as social work do not often correspond to the experiences and needs of women.

This text, *Relational Theory for Social Work Practice: A Feminist Perspective,* introduces social work professionals to relational theories, demonstrating how their basic tenets may be used in practice. Chapter One takes a longitudinal view of how the professional relationship has been conceptualized throughout the history of social work in the United States. Chapter Two explores how feminist thinkers, in developing their theory, built on ideas about the nature of the self that were formulated during the first 75 years of the twentieth century. Chapter Three focuses on the application of feminist relational concepts to the worker–client relationship. Chapter Four emphasizes the concept of mutual empathy and its central place in the feminist approach. Chapter Five examines relational processes, the structural components of relationship, and the implications of disconnection within the context of family, group, and community. Chapter Six presents a feminist view on the ethics and values of the profession, with a particular emphasis on the tension inherent in striking a balance between giving to others and giving to oneself.

Since relationships begin at birth and continue throughout the lifespan in different forms and with different subjects and objects, this book highlights the fact that connection and affiliative needs in human growth and behavior are critical throughout the life cycle. While men and women can both benefit from the concept of connection as primary over separation/individuation as a model for growth, women and men are socialized differently. Men frequently disavow their need for connection, often struggling for autonomy and independence while remaining unfulfilled, alone, and cut off from their authentic selves as well from the healing possibilities that relationship offers. Women, on the other hand, define their sense of self to a large extent within the context of their relational connections.

Relational ties provide a source of energy and a fuel for growth and development that continues to exert an influence on the individual's emotional and interactive life and make meaningful action in the environment possible. Thus, relational theory is an idea that has the potential to conceptualize the person within his or her environment. It is a theory that both supports and further develops the ecological systems perspective. I am referring not only to the one-to-one relationship, but also to the relationships established between clients and institutions. For example, when the parent of a child who is having difficulty navigating the educational system can form effective ties with school personnel, e. g., the teacher or the school social worker, that parent can help the child cope more successfully with the demands of the educational environment.

Throughout the history of social work, the individual and the environment have been artificially polarized, caught up in controversies such as cause versus function or the individual versus society. Relational theory respects and brings home the concept of self-determination in a way that may help people engage more actively to change themselves *and* make a positive impact on the world around them.

In the assessment as well as in the intervention phases of social work practice, we need to pay more attention to the client's relationship to his or her environment. When support is absent, when the client is socially isolated, is experiencing familial conflicts, or cut off from healthy relationships, he or she can experience depression, anxiety, and an overall sense of helplessness. A common solution is to further isolate oneself. I have found in my practice that when I focus on developing relationships as one of my goals with clients, this often leads to a change in the client's social and psychological functioning. It has always been my belief, particularly in my work with female adolescents, that one can only gain a clear and strong sense of self while simultaneously being *in* relationship with another. The social worker who is effective in helping clients negotiate distance and intimacy brings a substantial strength to his or her clinical practice.

Much of the evolving work in this area originated in publications from the Stone Center in Wellesley, Massachusetts, and has evolved as "self-in-relation" theory. Stone Center scholars include noted psychiatrist Jean Baker Miller, psychologists Irene Stiver and Janet Surrey, and social workers Julie Mencher, Wendy Rosen, and Clevonne Turner. Other feminist thinkers whose work has influenced this book include Jessica Benjamin, Nancy Chodorow, and Carol Gilligan.

While I learned a great deal in my doctoral program at Columbia University School of Social Work, the lesson that held the most relevance for me was a diagram that Dr. Carol Meyer used to depict the structure of an effective practice model. She pointed out that a sound conceptual approach to practice is built on knowledge, including theory and research, skills and intervention methods, and values, as well as on a world view which reflects how one perceives the human condition. The knowledge, skills, and values that underpin any practice method should have some degree of internal cohesion and integration. Furthermore, since the practice of social work requires thinking as well as doing, a sound theoretical base is essential. My intention in this book is to present a paradigm which melds feminist-relational theories with traditional social work theory to enhance practice.

In reviewing the traditional social work literature on practice and theory, I noticed that feminist theories—theories proposed by women or relevant to the female experience—receive scant attention. Although more recent social work volumes devote a page or two to some of the contemporary theories related to women (Berzoff , Flanagan, & Hertz, 2004; Cooper & Lesser, 2005; Kirst-Ashman & Hull, 2006), ), our knowledge base continues to be dominated by male theorists. How ironic this is for a female-dominated profession whose client population is predominantly female! And when social work authors do mention feminist theorists, such as Carol Gilligan, they are too often a mere "add-on" within a critique of the more widely espoused male theorists. Thus, my aim is to provide a text that more fully integrates a feminist-oriented relational perspective with practice; one that rests on a specific assumption that people are primarily motivated to form connections, and that the quality of relational ties with others are pivotal for adaptation and growth.

In its emphasis on the interactional elements of people's lives, a feminist-oriented relational approach is rooted in our professional history and harkens back to the settlement house days of Jane Addams. The method by which early social workers lived among urban settlers focused on connecting individuals to resources in the larger political and cultural system through the small group and local community. In her seminal 1934 monograph, *Between Client and Community*, Bertha Reynolds made explicit the importance of integrating giving help on an individual basis with community involvement and political awareness. When other psychiatrically trained workers like Reynolds were formulating individual treatment plans, the goals of which were to cure what was perceived as an illness residing in the individual, she articulated an approach to practice that addressed the need for the individual's adaptation to the community. This dual focus—on both the advancement of social justice and on individual adjustment—requires a theory that links the individual to the environment

The emphasis on relationship has not only been present from the very beginnings of our profession, it is also at its very heart. The relational emphasis is what istinguishes this discipline from all others. As highlighted in Chapter One, from the days of Mary Richmond, to the more psychiatric-minded social workers, to Helen Harris Perlman, the social work relationship has been seen as the connecting thread that links worker and client. In her book, *Relationship: The Heart of Helping People,* Helen Harris Perlman (1979) writes: "It is the theme and substance of this phenomenon we call 'relationship' that is a catalyst, an enabling dynamism in the support, nurture, and freeing of people's energies and motivations toward problem solving and the use of help" (p. 2).

One of the most important tools a worker has is the self. I wanted to present a book in which the worker is encouraged to use that self in a creative, authentic way. Workers who have a sufficient degree of self-awareness, who are able to work in the best interest of their clients, and who can move away from their own self-interest, should be encouraged to actively use their own feelings and thoughts and need not be afraid of relaxing ego boundaries. I wanted to present an approach that emphasizes realness and authenticity with clients while keeping in mind that the main concern is *the client's* best interest.

The challenge of this work is to not only combine acute self-awareness with a clear differentiation of self, but also to be able to emotionally connect with clients in a way that sensitively attunes to their thoughts and feelings. It is this dance of attunement that makes the social worker, at his or her best, a flexible, skilled instrument.

Reynolds (1951) emphasized that our practice is based in the world of social living whether we like it or not, and whether our theories correspond to it or not. Relational theory offers a concept of professional help that allows worker and client to share a common sense of humanity and for authenticity. Using her experience in the United Seamen's Service as a springboard, Reynolds championed a vision of people working together, leading to more social approaches to solving social problems. Let us not forget that social work is, first and foremost, a *social* profession—our history clearly speaks to this idea.

# Acknowledgements

I would like to acknowledge the invaluable assistance and editorial help from the following people:

Andrew Gottlieb
Andrea Raphael-Paskey
Marcy Bullmaster-Day
Stephanie Golden

I would also like to thank the following friends and colleagues who carefully reviewed sections of this book, edited case material, and made important suggestions (in alphabetical order):

Janet Bliss
Ilanna Dunner
Judy Fox-Fleisser
Arleen Maiorano
Claudine Schweber
Vicki Fern Taranto

I am also grateful to my friends and family who expressed much interest in my work and offered support and encouragement while I was engrossed inuring engrossment with this book—I am sure you know who you are.

I wish to recognize my colleagues in the Lehman College of the City University of New York Department of Social Work who embody the virtues of mutuality and collaborative respect. Special thanks go to Dr. Madeline Moran, Chair of the Department of Sociology, and Dr. Norma Kolko Phillips, Chair of the Department of Social Work.

I would also like to acknowledge my daughters, Melanie and Mandy, who make me proud of the young women they have become. And last but certainly not least I would like to thank David, who painstakingly read every page of this book and offered invaluable contributions.

# 1 The History of Social Work through a Relational Lens

Social work has long been concerned with relationships. Beginning in the last half of the nineteenth century in the pre-professional days of the Charity Organization Societies (COS), and continuing to the present, attention has alternated between the individual and the individual's relationships in his or her environment. Furthermore, the nature of the client–worker relationship and its function have shifted depending on prevailing economic, political, and social trends, such as the influences of Social Darwinism, Freud's psychoanalytic theory, advances in psychiatry and psychology, and wars and their aftermaths. This chapter will take a longitudinal view of how the social work relationship has been conceptualized and used. It will also examine how social work has dealt with the individual's relationships with friends, family, community and other social systems in the environment.

## Casework Before 1920: The Attempt to "Uplift"

Between the late 1800s and the early 1900s the Charity Organization Society (COS) movement came into prominence as a way of helping the poor by providing an alternative to public relief. The Charity Organization Societies were philanthropic organizations functioning under private auspices and endowed with a moral mission of moving the poor, intemperate, and indolent toward self-sufficiency and financial independence—a goal consistent with the spirit of individualism in a capitalist society. Partly a product of the era of Social Darwinism, which fostered a belief that those who could not manage in society without help were unlikely to survive, this ideal of helping people to become self-sufficient was carried out by the Societies' "friendly visitors" (Freedberg, 1984).

In keeping with the Judeo–Christian ideals of good citizenship, upper- and middle-class female volunteers acted as "friendly visitors" who, through face-to-face contact, attempted to uplift the mental and moral nature of the less fortunate and to motivate people applying for aid to find decent work and become good citizens. Occasionally charity workers also provided short-term financial assistance (Lubove, 1969). Boston COS leader Octavia Hill's (1875) motto "not alms but a friend" was reflected in the charity worker's new attitude of sympathy, rather than fear and pity, towards the poor and the adverse circumstances they had to overcome.

However, while visitors were instructed to form friendly relations with the applicants, in part to gain their cooperation, the disparity in social and economic power perpetuated a system of inherent paternalism that rendered the notion of "honest and simple" friendship somewhat paradoxical. The realization that the relations between visitor and client might not actually be "friendly," in the sense that they did not produce a basis for a satisfactory relationship, contributed to the decline of friendly visiting in the twentieth century and the move toward a more systematic method of helping the poor (Lubove, 1969). By the end of the 1800s, paid agents (usually men) had joined the ranks of the friendly visitors (usually women), and their strategies could be grouped into five areas representing the principles of what they called "scientific philanthropy": 1) investigation, 2) registration, 3) friendly visiting, 4) cooperation, and 5) constructive work. The major method of the Societies became systematic investigation into the causes of dependence and pauperism, in order to provide an individualized solution to the problems of the poor. As the nineteenth century drew to a close, charity giving was becoming more scientific and rational, heralding a new era of professionalization.

## The Professionalization of Social Work

Mary Richmond (1861–1928), a pioneer in the development of this new profession, helped shape American social work philosophy and practice during this period. By the turn of the twentieth century Richmond was established as a leader in the field, having been at the helm of two of the largest COSs in the country: the Baltimore Charity Organization Society (1891–1907) and the Philadelphia Charity Organization Society (1900–1905).

From the beginning of her career with the COS movement, Richmond recognized that relationship itself was a fundamental factor in the helping process. According to Richmond (1899), "Friendly visiting means intimate and continuous knowledge of and sympathy with a poor family's joys, sorrows, opinions, feelings, and entire outlook upon life" (p. 180). But this notion of the client–worker relationship was about to transform itself into a more "professional" one, in which the worker used him or herself as an instrument for change.

Richmond and her contemporaries, including Mary Jarrett and Ida Canon, all recognized the importance of placing a care-centered female relational field within a scientific framework of professional practice, both to legitimate themselves with respect to their client population, and to gain support from the male-dominated professions of medicine, psychology, and the natural sciences (Hiersteiner & Peterson, 1999).

By 1908, Richmond had moved away from her COS colleagues, whose focus had been on the moral roots of dependency, to a new concept of social work based on a scientific approach to casework. In 1909 she became the director of the Russell Sage Foundation's Charity Organization Department in New York, where she was able to devote herself to teaching and research (Pumphrey & Pumphrey, 1961).

Convinced that social work needed specific skills, knowledge, and a standardized, systematic method of practice that could be transmitted through formal training, Richmond called for the establishment of a school of "applied philanthropy." This was revolutionary, because women were not encouraged to undertake higher education in preparation of a paid career (Lubove, 1969). A one-year course was established at the New York School of Philanthropy in 1904 (later the New York School of Social Work and, since 1962, the Columbia University School of Social Work). Coinciding with the proliferation of schools of social work in the teens, the term "social worker" came into general usage (Ehrenreich, 1985).

Richmond, who was closely allied with the medical establishment in the Baltimore hospitals, applied the linear model of the medical sciences—diagnosis, treatment, cure—to social casework, the dominant method of social work activity in her time. In her groundbreaking book *Social Diagnosis* (1917), she introduced her method of casework practice, arguing that good social work was based on disciplined study and observation, a thorough gathering of social evidence, an interpretation of the data, an accurate diagnosis of the problem, and an appropriate treatment plan. By demanding a thorough and systematic gathering of facts, she believed, the social worker could uncover the cause of the problem and develop an eventual "cure" for the person in trouble (Germain, 1970). As part of her innovative systematic approach, Richmond (1917) understood the importance of relationships in assessing human behavior in the social environment. She describes "social diagnosis" as:

> the attempt to make as exact a definition as possible of the situation and personality of a human being in some social need—of his situation and personality, that is, in relation to the other human beings upon whom he in any way depends or who depended upon him, and in relation to the social institutions of his community.
>
> (p. 357)

By the time she wrote *Social Diagnosis*, Richmond had moved toward replacing the "friendly" relationship with the more formal expertise of a professional social worker trained in a systematic method of uncovering causes and treating the individual and family. Her focus on "action of mind upon mind" meant that while she described casework practice in terms of social investigation and the use of social evidence, she based her direct practice on the individual and his or her unique personal characteristics and difficulties.

In her major work, *What is Social Casework?* (1922), Richmond continued to highlight the individualized approach to social work, focusing on the client's ability to adjust to the objective realities in his or her life. This included the personal context of family, friends, and immediate neighborhood, as well as social relationships with community institutions such as the church, and with social service agencies. She defined the casework method as consisting of "those processes which develop personality through adjustments consciously effected, individual by individual, between men and their social environments" (pp. 98, 99). Although Richmond considered the social context beyond the individual and family in studying the individual, her actual practice side-stepped social reform and focused on a scientific method of study, diagnosis, and treatment, with the goals of individual change and social adjustment. Like the friendly visitor of the Charity Organization Societies, the social worker remained in control of the relationship. The difference was that in Richmond's configuration, the client was viewed as a diagnostic entity dependent on the social worker who, armed with expert knowledge, used him or herself as a professional tool to effect change within the individual (Ehrenreich, 1985).

It is important to note that, compared to the preconceived moral judgments about the character of the poor held by early COS workers, Richmond's objective approach to problem solving, which individualized each client's particular situation, was progressive for her time. The establishment of a professional client–casework relationship required objectivity; there was no room for moral judgment (Lubove, 1969).

## The Settlement House Era: Late Nineteenth to Early Twentieth Centuries

In addition to the COS movement, another group of concerned middle- and upper-class individuals sought to extend their help and their services to poor and working-class people in urban communities. The Settlement House movement began in large cities at the turn of the twentieth century, when social work was in transition from an avocation to a paid profession, and at a time when thousands of immigrants were arriving in America daily looking for opportunity and freedom in a newly prospering society. Housing, working conditions and sanitary conditions were poor, as immigrants making sub-standard wages crowded into tenements.

Reformers and Settlement House pioneers such as Jane Addams were concerned that these newcomers, who had no political power, were being manipulated for the good of local politicians. Furthermore, they feared that immigrants felt anonymous and disconnected from their new society. The Settlers believed that they could at least enhance neighborhood life and community relations so that relationships between the Settlers and residents would be more personal and representative of their interests. Thus, the bulk of Settlement work consisted primarily of progressive political activities, organizing for civic and community services and reforms, and small-group classes to educate newly arrived immigrants and to help them adapt to American cultural mores.

Unlike Richmond's early caseworkers, however, the Settlement workers wanted to carry out their mission in close relation to the people they served. Working side by side with community residents, these dedicated workers established relationships that involved doing *with*, rather than doing *for*, with the intention of promoting equality between themselves and community participants. Typically, they believed in what Jane Addams called the "reciprocal relationship of classes" (Smith, 1977). In their helping relationships, they modeled appropriate social roles and worked to develop interpersonal relationships into a mutual aid system (Wenocur & Reisch, 1989).

Addams, who believed that women should be active in community and political affairs, also saw Settlement House work as an outlet for women to extend their "natural" sense of maternal responsibility—the skills and values of motherhood—to disenfranchised and economically disadvantaged communities. Ironically, gender roles traditionally associated with the domestic sphere replicated themselves in relationships outside the home, perpetuating gender-linked stereotypes associated with the social work profession (Ehrenreich, 1985).

The Settlement House commitment to instructional and practical services, group activities, and social reform was the forerunner of the group-work method of the 1930s, 1940s and 1950s and the community action movement of the 1960s. Regardless of the specific approach—developmental, rehabilitative, recreational, or mutual aid—the group worker's prevailing consideration is to elicit common concerns, common interests, and common life situations, and to instigate group interaction so that members feel invested in each other and in the group. Boundaries between leader and group varied depending on the type of group, although the original premise of group work was to encourage a democratic process of group involvement, which means that the main source of growth resides within the member rather than the worker; the worker is more of a facilitator than an expert (Tropp, 1977).

## The Impact of Freud on Social Casework

Before World War I, social work had little awareness of Sigmund Freud, whose psychoanalytic theory had not strongly established itself on American soil. His theory began to receive widespread attention at a time when returning World War I veterans were suffering from war neurosis. Thus, a new need for psychiatrically trained social workers provided the impetus behind the opening of the Smith Training School for Psychiatric Social Workers in 1918.

By the 1920s and 1930s, Freud's theory of personality development had become increasingly influential in social work circles. Freud's theories (1923/1961) gave social workers a theoretical framework for analyzing unconscious inner needs, individual problems, and root causes of behavior heretofore missing from Richmond's sociologically oriented casework. Consequently, the Freudian model of the client–worker relationship defined problems largely in personality terms, with the emphasis on intrapsychic conflict and transferential aspects of relationships (Freedberg, 1984).

The professional relationship was relevant for Freud and his social work followers in terms of the "transference" phenomena—feelings clients had toward earlier significant figures in their lives that they unconsciously projected onto the social worker. The social worker's interpretations of the transference could provide the key that unlocked neurotic conflicts, furthering an understanding of emotional processes and helping clients see how they repeated these relational patterns in the present (Garrett, 1958). The client's positive or negative transference was a therapeutic issue especially when it interfered with the caseworker–client relationship and/or when it resulted in destructive behaviors in clients' lives (Family Service Society of America, 1958).

Freud's analysis of relationships beyond transference was basically limited to the child's primary relationship with the mother as the object of instinctually driven needs during the first four years of life. Moreover, the popularity of Freudian theory presented a dilemma for the social work profession—it was using a theory with a male-biased view of the sexes, focusing on the dynamics of male growth and conflict resolution, as a theoretical framework for a predominantly female profession with predominantly female clients. Freud seemed to feel that women were more passive than men and had more fragile ego boundaries. Translated into practice, Freudian theory did not provide a way to understand the specific issues and needs faced by female clients, specifically the growing desire for autonomy and power.

Freudian thinkers conceived of the individual psyche as an isolated entity only modestly influenced by the social group, its structures and processes. His model of the therapeutic relationship encouraged the worker to maintain an impassive self with rigid boundaries. Further, this relationship was cast as one-directional, leaving the social worker in control of the destiny of his or her clients. And, whereas social work increasingly began to regard effective social functioning as integral to its success, Freudian concepts encouraged a form of practice more intrapsychically oriented, leading the worker toward a form of practice detached from the community (Agnew, 2004). Nevertheless, Freudian theory did direct the social worker's interest toward individual problems and toward helping clients resolve conflicts in hopes of creating a more stable personality structure that would make possible more adequate adaptation to the environment.

## The Diagnostic School

The impact of Freudian psychoanalysis on social work theory in the 1920s and 1930s resulted in the development of the diagnostic school of social casework practice associated with such eminent scholar-practitioners as Gordon Hamilton, Fern Lowry, Lucille Austin, Annette Garrett, Betsey Libbey, and Grace Marcus (Minahan, 1986; Smalley, 1970). This phase of social work philosophy and practice, which spanned two world wars, was called the diagnostic school because of its stress on the importance of diagnosis in the treatment process. The diagnostic school furthered the development of casework as the dominant method in the field.

The diagnostic school viewed the therapeutic process as goal-directed and based upon the client's personality factors and social situation. The worker took responsibility for gathering data and evaluating individual capacities and limitations in order to arrive at therapeutic goals. Thus, on the basis of understanding the psychodynamics of the case, together with an assessment of the client's psychological status, the nature of the client's problems, and the social situation, a psychosocial diagnosis became the basis for intervention.

In a manner similar to that of Mary Richmond, the diagnostic school of social workers recognized the relationship as a conduit through which clients were guided in finding new ways of looking at themselves and their problems. This process was enhanced by a supportive worker, who could motivate the client toward accomplishing the treatment goal that best met that client's particular needs and diagnosis. The worker was there to listen and understand, and to help the client share life experiences and feelings in a way that might result in a reduction of tension and anxiety (Casius, 1950).

## The Functional School

During the late 1930s and early 1940s, a schism developed between case-workers who adhered to the diagnostic school and those who followed the functional approach to casework practice, which was based on Otto Rank's revolutionary concept of the will. Rank believed in the positive forces of human growth, with the person seen as an active agent in the areas of creativity and self-development. According to Rank, the individual development of self could best be understood as a balance of impulse, intellect, feeling and will. He placed particular emphasis on the individual will—a controlling, organizing force in the personality—and used this concept of will as a substitute for the ego.

Perhaps as a result of the sense of helplessness that many social workers felt during the Great Depression, Rank's optimistic view of humankind was much welcomed in the post-Depression era. The intent of the functional social worker was to move away from a deterministic Freudian interpretation of behavior in which the person was seen as driven by instinctual forces, to one in which the individual was deemed more in control of his or her life. Individuals' inborn will naturally moved them from an initial state of seeking union with significant others toward a state of individuation and autonomy in which they could eventually take over their own problem solving processes.

Rank's theory of personality and behavior held particular appeal for social worker Virginia Robinson and psychologist Dr. Jesse Taft, faculty members at the University of Pennsylvania School of Social Work, who saw the social work relationship as the core of all social work processes. Rather than trying to achieve any predetermined end based on an initial diagnosis, as in the diagnostic school, the functional school social worker used the relationship as a tool to help clients realize their own potential and reach psychological equilibrium (Robinson, 1930). According to Robinson, "engaging the other" through a professional social work relationship could release the growth potential inherent in all human beings, enabling clients to make and act on choices or decisions they identified as their own. The functionalists focused on the client's current situation as reflected in the relationship with the social worker, who carried out the function of the agency. The worker's use of agency function and structure and the purpose of the services being offered directed the helping process (Casius, 1950; Smalley, 1970).

In her landmark book, *A Changing Psychology in Social Casework* (1930), Robinson championed the use of the social work relationship as the primary tool of the social worker involved in a casework process oriented toward helping people make use of agency services in constructive ways (Smalley & Bloom, 1977). The social worker's competence and skills depended to a great degree on her self-development and self-awareness. The client's ability to engage in a growth-promoting relationship with a mature, self-aware worker could then be transferred to real-life situations in which new patterns of interacting with people in the environment could be established.

The following vignette illustrates how the diagnostic and functional approaches may be applied to practice. Mr. and Mrs. A. came to the Family Service Agency because of problems with their 10-year-old daughter, Janine. Janine, the eldest of four girls, is having the hardest time with the fact that Mrs. A. had breast cancer 18 months ago. Although her mother is now cancer free, Janine is very anxious about leaving Mrs. A. and frequently refuses to go to school. The social worker perceives the underlying cause of Janine's problematic behavior to be her separation anxiety since Mrs. A. was diagnosed with cancer. She is afraid her mother will die and is reluctant to leave her side.

A diagnostic school worker gathers as much information as possible on past history and present behavior to shed more light on the reasons for Janine's anxiety. The worker aims to gain a clearer understanding of the specifics of the mother–child relationship, the parents' attitudes toward Mrs. A.'s illness, their relationship, and Janine's early development, first by taking a history and then through observation. With the case worker's support and understanding, the therapeutic intervention begins with enabling Janine to talk about her fears and concerns about her mother's health. The worker is also concerned that the parents may be transferring their own anxiety onto

Janine and meets with them separately to help them talk about their feelings about the state of Mrs. A.'s health.

A worker guided by the functional approach spends more time reviewing agency services and functions. For example, the agency provides family counseling, family advocacy, and family-life education. The worker contracts with the client system and tries to help Janine and her parents decide how they can best utilize these services and benefit from the casework relationship. The social worker's activities might be directed toward helping the parents become better informed and self-directing so that they themselves can take more responsibility in helping Janine get to school. The worker models developmentally appropriate ways for Mr. and Mrs. A. to deal with Janine in the here-and-now.

The schism between the functional and diagnostic schools became more pronounced in the 1930s, when functional casework challenged Freudian concepts of therapy and placed its emphasis on time-limited treatment goals. Nevertheless, even though the functional school of thought emphasized agency function as the key to professional process, and the diagnostic school emphasized a linear model of assessment, the two approaches had more in common than their adherents may have realized. For example, in both schools the worker controlled the relationship, by virtue of either agency function or the worker's diagnosis.

## Development of Relational Perspective after World War II

After World War II, American social work philosophy and practice shifted more toward the relational perspective. In the late 1940s and the 1950s, efforts were made to bridge the gap between the functionalists and diagnostics, and greater attention was paid to clients' interactions with the social systems in their environment. Adapting psychodynamic ideas to a more social concept of casework, a group of eminent social work scholars and practitioners from the pre-war era, including Gordon Hamilton, Bertha Capen Reynolds, Florence Hollis, and Helen Harris Perlman, were instrumental in shaping the new American social work philosophy and practice.

Representing the diagnostic school, Gordon Hamilton saw the client–worker relationship as a way to strengthen and assess the individual's capacity to take action in relation to the environment. She expanded social work's unit of attention beyond the individual to include the impinging environment and the problem situation, which she termed the "person-in-situation configuration" (Germain, 1970; Hamilton, 1951). Reacting to the caseworker's bias toward the psychological aspects of practice, Hamilton's person-in-situation paradigm was an attempt to view both the inner psychological realities and the objective social context as one interrelated whole (Germain, 1970).

Thus, the objective of practice was to enable the individual to change, to bring about change in the situation, or both. Formulating the objective in this way led the worker to focus on the client's transactions with the social environment, such as the family, small group, and community (Hamilton, 1951). Like Mary Richmond, Hamilton emphasized the fact that the worker must individualize all aspects of the casework relationship. For example, two pregnant teen mothers may be facing the same economic and family difficulties, yet each might react differently to her situation; thus the social worker reacts differently as well. Or two pregnant teenage mothers may react in similar ways but be facing different economic and family difficulties.

For Hamilton, the concept of human relationships was fundamental in all social casework practice: the experience of having a friendly, interested worker listen attentively to one's troubles, not minimizing the difficulty, not criticizing or advising, tends to induce a warm response in the client, leading to a sense of being understood—the deepest bond in either a personal or a professional association.

Helen Harris Perlman (1979), noted for her problem solving method, also recognized the use of the helping relationship as basic to the casework process. In her book *Relationship*, she advises the reader that the function of a helping relationship is to help people cope with and solve their problems. She aptly states that "relationship is a human being's feeling or sense of bonding with another" (p. 23). When both individuals in the casework relationship interact with warmth, acceptance, and feeling, energy is freed up, generating the motivation toward problem solving and the use of help. Perlman's book is further evidence that the importance of the social work relationship, as well as the relationships people have with others in their life, was now widely recognized in mainstream professional circles.

Perhaps more than anyone, Bertha Capen Reynolds, practitioner, scholar, and activist, recognized the interdependence between the client and his or her social community. Having witnessed the contraction of democratic values and individual freedoms in Europe, she asserted the importance of establishing a social work relationship that made it possible to maximize a sense of equality between client and worker. Reynolds' perspective on relationships was as much a political and philosophical orientation as it was a practice principle. Delivering social work services in the personal social service department of the United Seamen's Service, she believed that because both client and worker were members of the same organization, a reciprocal relationship between the two was possible.

The personal social service department was set up in the hall of the National Maritime Union making it possible for her to work in proximity to the people social work served. Consistent with this philosophy, Reynolds placed the principle of client self-determination—the client's right to determine his or her own course of treatment—in the center of the social work process, freeing clients from the vestiges of any paternalistic relationship (Reynolds, 1951).

In the 1950s and 1960s the emerging concepts of social systems theory and ego psychology offered social workers new ways to understand the complex psychosocial phenomena behind human behavior, including relationships between people, social groups, and institutions. As a result, greater attention was paid to clients' interaction with the social systems in their environment.

Social systems theory is a way of thinking adapted from general systems theory, which views phenomena at all levels—human, plant, animal—as having common properties and principles. The basic idea is that each component of the system is simultaneously influenced by, and influences, the others. Systems theory made social workers more keenly aware of the fact that individuals are engaged in constant exchanges with other systems in their environment—especially other people.

Ego psychology, according to Edna Goldstein (1984), comprises a related set of theoretical concepts about human behavior that focus on the origins, development, structure, and functioning of the executive arm of the personality, the ego, and its relationship to other aspects of the personality and the external environments. Psychological concepts of the ego helped social workers focus on the adaptive capacities of the ego to cope with internal and external stress, and to form and sustain relationships.

In her book *Casework: A Psychosocial Therapy* (1981), Florence Hollis focused on "the treatment of individuals experiencing problems in their interpersonal relationships" (p. 3). Hollis saw the client–worker relationship as a microcosm through which to assess the difficulties clients might be having in other relationships in their lives. She emphasized the importance of the continuous interaction between inner psychological process and external social systems. In essence, Hollis elaborated on Hamilton's person-in-situation configuration to frame her psychosocial approach to casework.

However, even though Hollis's understanding of the client's reality included interpersonal transactions between individuals and social systems of varying sizes, her view did not have a major effect on practice. Interventions were still basically targeted at personality change, perhaps because influencing social relationships was a political issue that agencies did not have the power or authority to address (Germain, 1970).

In the 1960s, however, large-scale social change impacted the social work field and redirected attention to the social environment. The War on Poverty, the Economic Opportunity Act of 1964, the civil rights movement, and later movements for equality such as the women's movement inspired the launching of community action programs. These programs emphasized concrete services such as day care and health services, along with community participation, group methods, and advocacy. Community representatives were invited to sit on agency boards in policy making and advisory roles and sometimes were involved in planning and administering programs (Turner, 1977).

As Bertha Capen Reynolds had advocated, social work relationships became more mutual and participatory, with clients more invested in the services they received than in the previous casework era. In order to achieve social change, social workers set their sights on maximum participation of clients in planning for delivery of services. Working in partnership with community residents and consumers of services, social workers encouraged clients to have as much input as possible into the services they received.

Since the 1960s, social work has ventured in new directions, adding theoretical and practical approaches to its professional foundation. These new concepts and techniques include family theory and family therapy, crisis theory and crisis intervention, task-centered short-term work, couples counseling, self-help groups, and cultural and cross-cultural theories. It is time for the burgeoning body of feminist scholarship, which includes gender perspectives on human growth and behavior and a feminist relational approach to practice, to be fully integrated into the social work of the twenty-first century—taking us back to the mission described by the Settlement House Movement and by Bertha Reynolds—of providing services close to the people social work serves.

# 2 Relational Theory in a Nutshell

Feminist relational theory presents a new concept of the nature of the self, based upon its relationships with others. When incorporating a new approach to practice, it is helpful to examine the theoretical roots that gave rise to it and that support its clinical application. Accordingly, this chapter brings together a collection of theorists who share the view that 1) connections and affiliative needs are crucial to the growth and development of the self, and 2) the social organization of roles is different for men and women, which profoundly affects the quality and nature of their relationships. We will explore how, in developing their theories, these feminist thinkers built on theories about the nature of the self that were developed during the first three-quarters of the twentieth century and extended them in a new direction.

The early roots of a female relational/cultural perspective can be found in the work of Melanie Klein and Karen Horney, as well as in object relations theory, interpersonal psychoanalysis, and self-psychology. These last three approaches all share two features: 1) an emphasis on the client's sense of self and 2) an emphasis on the interaction between the individual and the object world—that is, the nature and qualities of this interaction with others as predictors of change.

## Klein and Horney

Historically, direct social work practice has incorporated the work of mostly male theorists into its knowledge base. In the 1920s and 1930s, neo-Freudian psychiatrists Melanie Klein and Karen Horney revised Freud's original theory, which was built on the concept of internal drives unrelated to the environment. Freudian theory and its derivatives presented an individualistic picture of human beings motivated by id-driven desires and needs, in which the primary goal of behavior is the attainment of gratification. In this model, the self is shaped not by mutually interacting relationships with others, but by relating to the other as an object whose sole purpose is to satiate one's impulses and gratify one's needs. As women, Klein and Horney understood the shortcomings of applying Freudian theory to female clients, and they interpreted psychoanalytic conflict within an interpersonal and cultural context. Although Klein and Horney gradually infiltrated the male-oriented psychiatric world of the 1920s and 1930s, and made major contributions to understanding human behavior and development, they were virtually ignored in mainstream social work circles.

Melanie Klein's concept of object-related drive theory emerged in the 1930s and expanded on Freud's drive model (Greenberg & Mitchell, 1983). Building on Freud's view that the infant is driven by basic biological impera-tives and drives, she broadened its scope to include the object world (that is, other people). Klein understood that drives were inherently connected to a complex web of objects in the environment, and therefore, intrinsically relational (St. Clair, 2004). Klein used the term *inner object* to suggest that there was no separation between infant and caretaker.

Klein's understanding of the inner world of the child gives insight into early dyadic relational processes, and provides a window from which to look into later relational conflicts and processes. However, while Klein attributed fundamental importance to the infant's first object relation—the mother's breast—feminist relational theorists note that object-relational needs are central throughout the life cycle and become a lifelong basis for personality development. The kind of interpersonal relationships offered to the child can help him or her to master a particular developmental stage, and can also provide the potential for a corrective interpersonal experience.

Writing from the 1920s through the 1940s, Karen Horney cast rela-tional processes beyond the dyadic encounter to include the larger social and cultural context. A critic of Freud's view of female sexuality, she challenged the well-accepted assumption of penis envy popular in the mainstream psy-choanalytic circles of her time. Rather than ascribe any sense of "envy" to a biological fate of circumstance, she attributed women's feelings of inferior-ity to their social subordination in an inherently male-dominated culture. As Juliet Mitchell notes, "according to Horney, libido was still biological, but any sense of anatomical inferiority resulted from a realistic appraisal of the power structure of social relations in the real world. If a little boy is adored by his family, his sister wants what he has, not the anatomical [thing] but the emotional gratification he experiences" (Lacan, 1985, p. 125). Thus, Horney and Klein shifted the focus of female problems from a biologically and sexually rooted neurosis to a concern with the psycho-social context of interpersonal relations.

## The Interpersonal School

About a decade after Horney and Klein presented their socio-cultural view of psychoanalytic theory, Harry Stack Sullivan challenged Freud's focus on intrapsychic processes, concentrating on the interpersonal context, in which personality is shaped and behavior takes place. For example, Sullivan (1940) posited that behavior that may seem meaningless when viewed as an individual response will take on new meaning when observed in an interpersonal context such as the family. In other words, according to Sullivan, personality does not reside in the individual mind. Rather, the relational matrix—past *and* present relationships—is the organizer of the self. Sullivan's concept of personality fits well with that of feminist relational theorists. He defines personality as "the relatively enduring pattern of recurrent interpersonal situations which characterize a human life" (p. xi).

As Sullivan developed his approach, he increasingly focused on anxiety as the motivating force in the way the individual shapes his or her experiences in the world (Mitchell & Black, 1995). According to Sullivan, if anxiety is present in the "mothering" of the infant, the young child will look for a secure base to reduce the tension associated with the anxiety that the mother, or mother substitute, has induced. Subsequently, interactions that an individual feels as painful or threatening, based on his or her previous interpersonal experiences, will continue to drive behavior. On the other hand, social interaction that provides a secure base can release the person from anxiety. Thus for Sullivan, the personal relationship between therapist and patient is a critical determining factor in the outcome of treatment.

Sullivan's concept that the self is constituted through relationships with others is an important precursor of feminist self-in-relation theory. He reaffirmed the belief that the human being is inextricably linked to others in a series of interpersonal fields and that the need for soothing social relations continues to evolve throughout the life cycle. The questions for the social worker are: what kind of human interactions keep the person locked into nonproductive habits, and what can be done to change these patterns? The objective reality of one person's experience with another is not as important as what this experience subjectively means to the client (Mitchell & Black, 1995).

## The Object Relations School

Beginning in the 1940s and 1950s, the British and American "object relations" school of psychology gained popularity in the social sciences. It included different approaches to understanding people's interpersonal relations with the object world. The term "object," a technical word originally coined by Freud to refer simply to "that which will satisfy a need," was broadened to refer to the significant person or thing that is the object or target of another's feelings or drives (St. Clair, 2004). The emerging object relations school contributed a great deal to social work's understanding of child and human development and ways of adapting to the social environment (Mitchell, 1988).

British psychoanalyst John Bowlby (1969) believed that individuals are motivated not by drives but by forming attachments to other persons from the moment of birth. He defined attachment theory as a way of understanding human beings' propensity to create strong emotional bonds to significant others and of explaining the many forms of personality disturbance and distress that occur after separation and loss. Bowlby emphasized the survival function of attachment in enhancing safety through the infant's proximity to the caregiver. He saw attachment as an inborn, instinctive mechanism that is ascendant in the earliest years, the most critical and vulnerable time in the infant's life.

Drawing on a wide range of ethnological studies of instinctive behavior, Bowlby (1969) considered attachment behavior similar to imprinting in the animal species and necessary for survival. Attachment motivates the child to move toward a care-giving figure for protection, warmth, nurturing, and social interaction, in addition to feeding. The physical goal of proximity for survival is later supplanted by the more psychological goal of feeling close to the caregiver, whose responses strongly influence the child's present and future behavior patterns and personality states (Fonagy, 2001). Bowlby argued that the infant's attachment to the mother is a precondition for the satisfaction of all other needs, making her a primary object of importance (Mitchell, 1988).

Object relations theorists also contributed a great deal to social work's understanding of people's adaptation to the social environment. Scottish psychoanalyst W.R.D. Fairbairn constructed a model of object relations that was perhaps more psychological and less biological than those of any of his neo-Freudian counterparts. Like Klein, he believed that the ego and object are inseparable. Unlike Klein, he argued that the ego has its own source of energy, separate and apart from instinctual impulses, and organizes itself as a consequence of the accumulated quality of its relations with external objects during the first year of life. He argued further that the infant is oriented toward others from the beginning, not just to relieve frustration, but to establish an emotional bond with an external object.

Thus, the essential principle in Fairbairn's structural system is that the human being is essentially relation-seeking. Propelled by its own source of energy, the self or ego seeks out and maintains an intensive emotional bond with an external object throughout life (Kernberg, 1976).

Typically, object-relations theorists trace the trajectory of normal development as a movement from an infantile dependence on a part object (the mother's breast) to a mature dependence on a whole object (a whole person). Growth moves from an infantile attitude of taking to a more mature attitude of mutual giving and receiving between two differentiated individuals (St. Clair, 2004).

From the 1930s to the 1960s, D.W. Winnicott represented a new voice in the British object relations school. He devoted much of his attention to areas of child development, especially the mother–child interaction. Winnicott emphasized two key concepts that are relevant to social work's dual focus on the person and the environment: 1) the facilitating or holding environment, with its focus on adaptation, and 2) the "good-enough" mother, with its focus on the parent's proper attunement to the infant's needs and wants. Both terms describe parental figures giving themselves over to the child and reducing to a minimum frustration that the infant cannot manage on its own.

Winnicott linked the development of a healthy sense of self to specific qualities of the "good-enough" mother (Mitchell, 1988). Using this concept as an overarching theme, he invoked the idea of a reasonably empathic mother who is attuned to her infant's basic social-emotional and survival needs. The "facilitating" environment provided by this "good-enough" mother represents her effort to shape the environment around the child's wishes and to intuit what the child needs and wants. Winnicott places much importance on ego relatedness. Basic relational experiences are primary throughout life. In fact, primary relationships create experiences that provide for a sense of self—feelings of belonging, of being understood, accepted, and loved (Guntrip, 1971).

Winnicott's ideas hold meaning for the social worker in her efforts to shape the interpersonal environment around the client's needs and wants. The idea is for client and worker to build together a subjective sense of reality mediated by the relationship with a caring, empathic "mother" figure—the worker. As Applegate (1993) states, "Winnicott keeps the relationship in the spotlight, regardless of the intervention" (p. 5). However, like Klein's, Winnicott's theories are still anchored in Freud's instinctual model, in which pleasure from need-satisfaction forms the basis of relationship.

## Self-Psychology

The relational theories rest upon the premise that people have a powerful tendency to repeat basic relational patterns from their early years into the later stages of life. In the view of self-psychologist Heinz Kohut, the self develops out of interaction with certain key nurturing figures that he terms *selfobjects* (Fonagy, 2001). These selfobjects do not simply gratify the infant's biological needs and desires, but provide key functions that strengthen and support the development of a more realistic and positive sense of the self in the growing child. These selfobject functions may comfort, control tension, and help maintain stability of the self-system (Greenberg & Mitchell, 1983). The infant internalizes these functions as a way to strengthen its own growing sense of self and regulate its self-esteem. A simple example would be the way in which a person learns to cope with disappointment and loss at an early age.

Kohut emphasizes two distinct selfobject functions in his self-psychology: *Mirroring* takes place in a nurturing context in which the infant can begin to feel more known, more real, and more internally substantial. The maternal figure is responsive to the infant and reflects back enthusiasm, approval, and praise that reinforce the infant's spontaneously arising healthy narcissism. For example, the caretaker can respond with a loving smile, a proud gaze, or a soothing touch. In *idealizing*, the infant needs to form an idealized image of at least one parent and experience a sense of merger with this idealized selfobject. By feeling an essential likeness with the much-admired, omnipotent parent, the immature self feels stronger and more powerful (Mitchell & Black, 1995).

In the context of these two functions, the child experiences the mother's pride or disinterest as the acceptance or rejection of his or her active self. It is normal and necessary for a child to seek confirming, approving responses from a mother figure; our pursuit of recognition and attention offsets some of the loneliness and desire for closeness we feel throughout life. Like Sullivan, Kohut believes that individuals require a milieu of empathically responding selfobjects throughout their lives to gain recognition and attention. If we do not experience warmth and closeness, it is difficult to remain an active agent in any aspect of life.

The existence of selfobject functions implies that a reasonably integrated parent can meet the developmental needs of the infant and provide him or her with permanent psychological structures that serve to regulate tension and anxiety and to guide the child through different stages of self-development. Of course, the parent must feel self-confident and secure, so that the child can take in these soothing characteristics. When the parent possesses these qualities, selfobjects can provide for self-regulation and self-confidence, facilitating the development of a cohesive self that reappears in different forms throughout our adult years (Fonagy, 2001). Over time, the child will hopefully outgrow most of the need for an idealized and mirroring selfobject. This never fully happens. The need for an idealized and mirror selfobject continues throughout the life cycle.

Kohut assumes that most individuals are born into a responsive human milieu. However, this is not necessarily the case, and relatedness with others, a condition necessary for psychological survival, cannot be taken for granted. If parents' needs are unmet, it is harder for them to be appropriately responsive to the child (Rowe & Mac Isaac, 1991). This suggests that in order to help the child, the social worker must first help the parent to repair early deprivations or trauma.

Kohut's psychology of the self has profound implications for the worker–client relationship, in that he emphasizes empathic sensitivity to the patient's subjective experience and recognition of the need for life-long selfobjects. This focus raises the question of whether the worker can function as a positive selfobject for individuals who lack a stable sense of self, and identity and are vulnerable to sudden losses of self-esteem. Alternatively, can the social worker help the client seek new selfobject functions in the present environment, in the form of nurturing figures or caregivers, to compensate for earlier deficits?

Kohut's belief that personality disorders can be attributed to early deficits in selfobject introjections suggests that the clinician can compensate for less than adequate early relationships—at least to some degree—by creating an empathic, accepting environment where the worker is tuned into the client's needs and wants. In addition, there is the potential for new concepts of self and new value systems to be formed through favorable interactions with other sensitive, caring, and validating persons in the environment. Basing clinical work on the understanding that the relationship between client and worker permits new object relations to form thus reinforces the value social work has placed on the helping relationship (Mitchell, 1988).

One thing Kohut did not express an interest in, but which is important in a feminist relational approach, is the "other" who provides the selfobject function for the self. The feminist relational approach sees this other as a separate subjective being, which is what makes possible the inter-subjective mutuality involved in a give-and-take relationship. The use of the word "selfobject" still casts the "other" as an object gratifying the needs of the self, as opposed to expressing the idea that both parties are involved in mutual receptivity and affected by each other's actions (Jordan, 1991b).

The approaches described so far provide an underpinning for feminist relational theories. However, although these male-oriented structural relational theorists depart from traditional psychoanalytic thinking in their acknowledgment that autonomy from the object is not the primary mark of the healthy personality, by and large their work remains one-directional. By contrast, feminist theories emphasize the life-long centrality of relationships and assert that in mature dependence, the emphasis shifts from taking to giving, so that eventually a mutual exchange takes place.

## Infant Developmental Research

Any new theoretical paradigm for practice must rest on research-based propositions, and infant researcher Daniel Stern's (1985) work contributes more to modern-day feminist relational theory than that of perhaps any other developmental researcher/theorist. Stern's work brings attention to the fact that reciprocal interactions begin at birth. In *The Interpersonal World of the Infant*, Stern describes his research on the infant's subjective experience, focusing on the interaction and mutual regulation of babies and their primary caretakers. He hypothesizes that the infant forms his or her subjective sense of self in relation to another from the very beginning of life. For example, at the end of the first week of life, Stern argues, the mother's face has become a familiar perceptual gestalt and the infant can distinguish the smell of his or her own mother from that of others, indicating that the infant can conceive of another outside his or her self-boundaries. Each side of the mother–infant dyad complements the other; one person performs an action and the other receives it. Stern's work fits well with the female-oriented relational/cultural model approach presented in this book, in which the basic units of analysis are the bi-directional relational bonds and the relational matrix they form.

In reviewing Stern's research, in which he observed newborns interacting with their primary caretakers, we are reminded that this relational matrix begins to take shape much earlier than object relations and developmental theorists imagined. Stern's assertion that the early formation of a sense of core self is developed in interaction with the primary caretaker during the first month of life infers that the infant does not enter the world in a state of undifferentiated fusion, as object-relations theorists Margaret Mahler and others (1975) believed, but rather that the infant comes into the world with a cognitive awareness of himself or herself as distinct from others. Thus, Stern's basic organizing perspective places the relational self at the center of development from the moment the infant is born and asserts that this self is in a constant state of elaboration and reorganization throughout life.

According to Stern (1985), different senses of self emerge with the development of new capacities, the first being the core sense of self. At each major shift in maturation, there is a change in the subjective experience of the interaction between infant and caregiver, giving the infant increasing control over social interactions. For example, the infant takes part in regulating the level of excitement caused by the outside world by using gaze aversion to cut out stimulation that has risen above an optimum range. The caretaker, in turn, regulates her responses to adjust to the infant's stimuli barrier. With this kind of mutual regulation, the infant gains experience with self-regulation in response to the caregiver's sensitivities and ability to help the infant experience some control over the environment (Fonagy, 2001).

Stern's work suggests that a major task for the individual is to create increasingly complex and intimate ties with others while at the same time perceiving him or herself as having a self that is separate from the other. In other words, the process of development does not involve merger at one pole versus differentiation at the other, but rather the ability to balance the development of a separate self with the awareness and experience of interacting with another, that makes for a healthy personality.

Stern's work also indicates that an individual has a degree of mastery over his or her environment from the earliest days. Thus, the worker can assume that there is the potential for self-mastery even in clients who do not seem to have any sense of control over their lives. An informed relational social worker can therefore help the client engage in mutually regulatory relationships in which she or he feels a sense of control as opposed to helplessness.

Through repeated observations of mother–infant interactions, other infant–parent researchers, such as Beatrice Beebe and Frank Lachmann (2002), have also demonstrated that parent–child behavior does not operate in a unidirectional fashion. Rather it is a dyadic system characterized by mutual and reciprocal social exchanges over time. Each response by parent or infant triggers specific behavior in the other, resulting in a continuous feedback loop (Brazelton, Koslowski, & Main, 1974). These interacting behaviors form patterns that affect the nature of a person's relationships throughout life. This concept suggests the value of creating new opportunities for relationships that allow individuals to experience themselves differently. Like the parent, the social worker's role can be to interpret the client's signals and attune his/her specific responses to meet the client's needs.

This approach not only fits well with the principles of social systems theory, predominant in the teachings and practice of social work, but also underpins the feminist relational/cultural model of practice. Building on infant studies, feminist relational theories recognize that having an impact on another is a lifelong need (Reiter, 1995).

## Intersubjective Theory

The relational theorists affiliated with the Jean Baker Miller Institute at Wellesley College credit Robert Stolorow and the intersubjective theorists as having a major influence on their work. According to Stolorow and his colleagues (1994), a person's primary experience of self, self-esteem, and personality has its origins in the degree to which mutual regulation exists in the subjective world of the child–primary caretaker system. This intersubjective world includes shared ideas, emotions, impressions; it places the psyche in the realm of interacting human systems. An important indicator of well-being is the subjective reality of how the client experiences relationships and events.

Intersubjective theory fits well with systems theory and a feminist relational paradigm since it frames psychological phenomena in a broad interactional context and focuses on the reciprocal influences people have on one another. Simply stated, if a teenager is pregnant and does not feel supported, appreciated, or understood by her partner, or if that partner does not feel understood or supported by his family, it will be difficult for the teen to nurture her infant.

## Relational Theory from a Feminist Perspective

Relational theory from a feminist perspective is fully compatible with the core principles and values of direct social work practice. It provides a contextual relational view of self that is consistent with the person-in-situation ecological systems perspective of social work. This school of thought advances understanding of the emotional, social, moral, and cognitive development of women in particular. While most developmental theories devised by men emphasize the importance of disconnection from early relationships to achieve a separate self, women's experience in large measure, contradicts such theory and suggests that a new model of development is needed.

Traditional theories of human growth and development have usually relied on research using male subjects conditioned by the male experience in a Western industrialized society (Erikson, 1950; Levinson, 1978; Kohlberg, 1981). Based on cultural standards and expectations, which included ideals of competition, individual mastery, and independence, growth and development were expected to evolve out of a dyadic relationship with the primary caretaker through increasing levels of separation and personal individuation (Erikson, 1968; Mahler, Pine, & Bergman, 1975). Applying these principles of male development, which emphasize separation and independence, to women made them seem deficient rather than merely different.

The feminist relational approach emphasizes the nature and quality of connectedness to others. According to Janet Surrey (1991), early self-representations characterized by clear but flexible boundaries cohere around specific interactions with the primary nurturing figure and contribute to the development of a "relational self" in women. Counter to the traditional bias that suggests aspects of self unfolding along a developmental line of increasingly autonomous functioning, separation, and independence, Surrey argues that the self develops its structure in the presence of a finely tuned, shifting balance of connection and differentiation with significant others. In other words, she shifts the emphasis from separation and individuation to relationship with differentiation as a goal for healthy functioning. This model might be expressed as: *Rather than separate completely from you, I am going to define who I am in relation to you. Interaction with you allows me to get a better sense of myself than I could get on my own, so I'm going to stay connected to you.* Thus, relational theory allows us to appreciate the relational nature of women's sense of self, rather than judging their identity formation as deficient or lacking in some fundamental way.

Relational theory asserts that individual development actually proceeds by means of affiliation for both men and women. Men, however, are pressured by social sanctions to cut off from the other (usually a female figure) in the early years of life in search of a "masculine" identity. As a result, they may see relationship as a threat to their autonomy, success, and sense of self.

Building on the work of the theorists presented thus far, Stone Center leaders Jean Baker Miller, Alexandra Kaplan, Judith Jordan, Irene Stiver, Janet Surrey, along with their associates Carol Gilligan, Nancy Chodorow, Mary Belenky, and Jessica Benjamin, note the failure of traditional theories of human development to appreciate the relational nature of women's sense of themselves. As a paradigm for the study of all self-in-environment experience, these women posit an interactive sense of self, sometimes called "self-in-relation." In essence, the common organizing principle in this approach to clinical work is to give primacy to the capacity for, and continuity of, relationships in women's ordinary life experiences. For social work practice, the pathway toward development of a healthy sense of self includes helping the client reach increasing levels of choice, complexity, and satisfaction in her constellation of relationships.

Carol Gilligan (1982) is one of the first feminist theorists to note that the discrepancy between women's experience and the prevailing theories of human development was generally considered to represent a problem in women's development. Rather, according to Gilligan, what is missing from those theories is the idea that the development of the self and morality takes place within relationships and is embedded in a relational context that changes over time.

In her seminal book, *In a Different Voice*, Gilligan uses Lawrence

Kohlberg's theory of levels of moral development to make her argument that women fare less well than men in traditional theories of psychological and moral development. Kohlberg's theory, which centers on the development of what he calls a "justice" perspective, attributes a higher level of maturity to individuals who make moral decisions in accordance with their own sense of what is right, independently of others. Gilligan maintains that this approach does not accurately reflect women's development and experiences across the life cycle—experiences that socialize women to make decisions in line with their sense of caring for others. Her attempt to correct the male bias in Kohlberg's theory gave impetus to the development of her relational ethics of responsibility and care.

Gilligan's relational theory of responsibility and care represents an attempt to re-conceptualize the relationships between judgment and action, thought and experience, concepts of self and morality, and experiences of conflict and choice. She describes women as tending to hear a "different voice" than men when thinking through personal moral decisions. After extensive empirical observations of different ways in which women think about rights and responsibilities, Gilligan found that women's experiences and perspectives, and their overriding concern with relationships and responsibilities, affect their decision-making processes in myriad ways.

Women's differing concepts of self and differing behaviors reflect different kinds of judgments than those made by the males studied by Kohlberg. Women's experiences reveal that they learn about the world in relation to others, basing their decisions on feeling and a sense of care as well as on intellectual reasoning. Women are thus more likely to equate morality with helping and pleasing others than with the inclination, characteristic of men, to make decisions and moral judgments in terms of an abstract principle of justice.

Like Gilligan, psychologist Nancy Chodorow (1978) illustrates the difference between developmental pathways for boys and girls. Since the majority of primary caregivers for young children in our society are women, it is natural that boys and girls will be affected differently in their personality formation and gender identity development, beginning as early as the pre-oedipal stage. Using object-relations and psychoanalytic theory, Chodorow describes how girls internalize aspects of mothering—care, empathy, and softness, for example—in their identification with their same-sex parent. These traits are re-enacted with their own children and are eventually reproduced psychologically and sociologically across generations.

Boys, by contrast, usually have an opposite-gender caregiver and may feel socially coerced to sever their pre-oedipal ties to their mothers in order to develop a sense of self and individuate out of relationship. Thus, ego boundaries become more rigid in boys than girls in an effort to protect and secure their masculine identity (Chodorow, 1978).

A great deal can be learned about growth-enhancing interactions from studying women's experiences, since women's sense of self is, to a great extent, organized around being able to make and then maintain affiliation and relationship. Women have been placed in a subordinate position precisely because of this concern with building relationship and their associated role of serving others, both of which our culture devalues. This power dynamic trickles down to theory building; pejorative terms such as merger, dependency, and fusion have been used to characterize the child's early relationship with the mother, while separation and independence are designated as key criteria of mature psychological development.

In her ground-breaking book *Toward a New Psychology of Women* (1976), Jean Baker Miller lays the groundwork for a feminist relational perspective on practice. She argues that power inequality in male and female gender roles relegated females to a subordinate position vis-à-vis males in this society, and suggests that, to the extent to which mutually enhancing interactions are unlikely in situations of unequal power, growth may require recognizing difference and openly engaging in conflict. This does not mean that relational ties must be severed—rather, they need to adapt to complex maturational, social, and developmental processes, have flexible boundaries, and be open to change.

Miller posits that the role, function, and social situation of women in a male-dominated society—in other words, the social structuring of gender relationships—is intricately connected to understanding the development of mind, identity, and self. Like Gilligan and Chodorow, Miller argues that women develop a sense of self in a context of attachment and affiliation with others, while most men build their identity through increasing levels of autonomy and separation. Thus, the female sense of self becomes organized to a considerable extent around being able to make, and then maintain, affiliations and relationships. For example, it is much more likely that a woman who is depressed is suffering from the loss of affiliation with others than that a depressed man will be suffering from such a loss. He may be suffering from the loss of a job or some other status symbol that reflects society's affirmation of his manhood.

In the mid-1980s, using Miller's work as a springboard, theoreticians, researchers, and clinicians at the Stone Center for Developmental Services and Studies at Wellesley College began their pioneering efforts to create a new model of psychological development for women. Originally termed "self-in-relation theory" by Miller, the model emphasizes the fact that, for women, the core sense of self is organized, developed, and maintained in the context of important relationships throughout life (Surrey, 1991). Miller (1991a) refutes traditional developmental theorists, such as Erikson and Mahler, who view ego development as a process of separating oneself out from the matrix of a "fused" existence with another. Instead, Miller suggests that from the moment of birth, the development of an internal representation of self takes place in active interchange with other selves—what she calls "being in relationship." Miller proposes that the infant begins to be and act like the main caregiver, identifying not only with the caregiver as "some static figure described only by gender, but with what the person is actually doing" (p. 3). Thus, the infant begins to develop an internal differentiated representation of himself or herself within close connection to another within the first few months of life:

> The child experiences a sense of comfort only as the other is also comfortable, or, a little more accurately, as they are both engaged in an emotional relationship that is moving toward greater well-being.
>
> (p. 3)

The movement toward mutuality is central to successful coping and healthy development. As Judith Jordan (1991d) eloquently states:

> Movement toward mutuality lies at the heart of relational development. Rather than viewing people as primarily motivated by a need for self-sufficiency and personal gratification, a relational perspective acknowledges our deep need to establish connections with other people.
>
> (p. 1)

In relationships characterized by mutuality, individuals relate to one another based on an interest in each other as whole, complex persons and with an awareness of the other's subjective experience. In such an exchange, one both affects the other and is being affected by the other; one extends oneself out to the other and is also receptive to the impact of the other (Jordan, 1991b).

In essence, the emphasis on mutuality proposes a major paradigm shift in Western psychology as a whole: from a psychology of the separate self to a psychology of relational being. Jordan (1997a) traces several biases in the traditional view of the self, such as its emphasis on the self as a bounded, discrete, decontextualized entity, to influences from psychoanalytic theory and to the socio-political context of the Western industrialized world, which idealizes that view of the self. She asserts that, to gain authority, psychology as a discipline has modeled itself on the "hard" sciences (such as physics) rather than being seen as an extension of a humanistic tradition associated with female sensibilities. She writes: "Newtonian physics posited discrete, separate entities existing in space and acting on each other in predictable and measurable ways. This easily led to a study of the self as a comparably bounded and contained 'molecular entity' " (p. 10).

This inner conviction of the "separate self" erects rigid boundaries between subject and object, according to Jordan (1991a). These boundaries act as a barrier that prevents sharing and understanding the momentary psychological state of another person, making fluid interchanges between people difficult. The concept of empathy—the dynamic cognitive process of joining with and understanding another's subjective experience—is central to Jordan's intention of altering the traditional boundaries between subject and object and promoting an inter-subjective notion of relationship.

Like Stolorow and Jordan, Jessica Benjamin (1988) articulates a theory of "inter-subjectivity" that questions the tendency in psychoanalytic thinking to polarize the child as the "subject" and the mother as the "object." Instead, Benjamin re-conceptualizes the psychic world as "a subject meeting another subject" (p. 20). She refutes the notion of traditional object-relations theorists that mother and infant are merged at birth. Instead, she develops a feminist orientation, asserting that the self develops its structure in the presence of a shifting balance of connection and differentiation. Self-representations characterized by clear but flexible boundaries and appreci-ation of difference from important others exist alongside self-representations in which self and other overlap.

Simply stated, people influence each other. Each party in a relational interchange must be capable of recognizing the subjective feelings, rights, and experiences of the other, in order to have a meaningful experience in the other's presence. Actualizing this capacity for mutual recognition—that is, taking into account the subjectivity of the other—can enable all individuals to function optimally (Benjamin, 1995).

In the early 1990s, the self-in-relation model was renamed the Stone Center Relational/Cultural Model to emphasize the fact that psycho-social development takes place in and through increasingly complex cultural, social, and relational contexts (Miller & Stiver, 1997). Though much atten-tion has been given to relational processes that occur between two or more people, the relational/cultural approach asserts that variables such as gender, class, ethnicity, and sexual preference—in fact the entire context in which societies are organized—have a major impact on the experiences of everyday relationships. Thus, the relational/cultural perspective embraces a political and economic analysis of patriarchy.

The Stone Center Model views connections, disconnections, and re-connections in relationships as core developmental processes throughout life. It posits that optimally: 1) we grow in, through, and toward relationship, 2) for women, especially, connection with others is central to psychological well-being, and 3) movement toward relational mutuality can occur throughout life, through mutual empathy and responsiveness (Jordan, 1997a; Kaplan, 1991b; Miller & Stiver, 1997; Spencer, 2000; Surrey, 1991).

A feminist relational paradigm for practice creates a framework for exam-ining the interaction between cultural imperatives and interactive systems at different levels; family, organization, community, etc. Along with this set of cultural role expectations, politics, social privilege, as well as economic and class restrictions, affect people's psycho-social functioning. Many women experience a sense of oppression as a result of having accepted and internal-ized the cultural devaluation of their experiences and the perceived limita-tions in their development. The practitioner can raise the consciousness of both female and male clients by clarifying the cultural norms surrounding the notions of "masculinity" and "femininity" in our society.

A feminist relational approach to practice emphasizes mutuality and empathy—that is, gaining insight into the subjective reality of the client without any judgment or pre-conceived notions about behavior. The participants are equal partners, each allowing himself or herself to be affected by the other. Thus, the worker is committed to sharing her thoughts, feelings, and knowledge, and is willing to be affected by the client. Whether in the worker–client relationship, or in relationships with significant (and not so significant) others, the capacity to see the other as a person separate from yourself, who does not exist solely to gratify your needs, who experiences her own stresses, feelings, and mind states, is essential for creating successful, cooperative relationships based on mutual respect and understanding.

# 3 The Client–Worker Relationship

This chapter focuses on the use of feminist relational concepts in the client–worker relationship. Since social work's mission involves change, this would include finding new ways to use the professional relationship that moves clients out of their isolation, out of destructive relationships, and into connections that are healthier and more growth producing. Not only are social workers uniquely positioned to create the kinds of relationship that enhance self-esteem and mobilize client strengths, but we can also observe and assess clients' relationships with other social systems, such as school personnel, work colleagues, neighbors, and extended family.

There are many different types of relationships in individuals' lives, the client–worker being just one prototype of what a relationship can be. Guided by the Stone Center *Works in Progress* series, the feminist relational model requires the worker to focus attention on the client's relational processes, the structural components of relationships and the implications of chronic disconnection. As suggested by Nancy Chodorow (1978), an inner sense of connection to others is a central organizing feature in women's development. Social and cultural mores have made it easier for females to seek out relationships and to stay connected longer than males. However, the internalized gendered world is not fixed, and the desire for connection can cut across gender lines, particularly in today's changing society.

A feminist relational viewpoint places emphasis on relational yearnings as normative, not only connected to unresolved residues of childhood, as some psychodynamic theorists have argued (Greenberg & Mitchell, 1983). Since we all replay significant relational dynamics, the potential power in the therapeutic relationship lies in the opportunity to provide the client with a reparative experience. This relationship can then serve as a model for other relationships—ones in which the client can both reshape internal negative images resulting from past hurt, and reconstruct other relationships in more positive ways. This desire for relationship, considered to be a life-long motivating force that drives feeling, thought, and action, reinforces the importance social workers have given to a dynamic systems approach, in which the emphasis is on interaction. Beebe et al. (2002) documented infants as young as three months adjusting their behavior to their mothers' movements, supporting the notion of interaction as continuous and mutually constructed, a reciprocal form of attunement people engage in throughout life.

The therapeutic goal is to create a deeper, more meaningful sense of connection between worker and client and between client and others. An authentic and responsive relational context characterized by mutuality, reciprocity, and intersubjectivity has the potential to enhance clients' capacity to cope under adverse circumstances and to promote adaptation under normative ones. The energy of the client–worker relationship can become the fuel for decision-making that enhances clients' ability to take action. Simply put, social workers are change agents, and relationships marked by mutuality can facilitate the helping process. Social workers can also be role models who help people learn how to relate to others in healthier ways. Just as mothers and fathers are not born knowing how to parent but must learn these skills through practice, so people learn how to relate to others through modeling, identification, and education.

Exploring all of the client's relationships—present *and* past—may prove highly significant in understanding them. For example, a father who abandoned his child years ago and so is not present in the child's day-to-day life may be *the* most important variable to consider when working with that child and his or her family. Yet the inexperienced social worker may overlook this.

## The Social Work Relationship: Traditional Approaches, Contemporary Trends

While relationship has been traditionally defined as the basic condition in which two or more people with some common interest connect, the advent of globalization and increased immigration make it increasingly important for social workers to learn to relate to clients with greater cultural sensitivity. Concepts such as dependency, use of self, transference-counter-transference, and boundaries as traditionally interpreted may no longer fit the diverse populations with whom we work.

### The Client–Worker Relationship

The role of the client–worker relationship has long occupied a prominent position in direct social work practice, particularly in casework, which dominated the field from the 1920s through the 1960s. In many ways the rise of professionalism has been a double-edged sword. On the one hand, social work practice has been better informed and elevated in terms of professional status. On the other hand, the professional relationship can feel unnatural without some degree of genuineness and spontaneity.

Virginia Robinson (1930) credited the client–worker relationship with the ability to provide internal support needed to bolster ego functions and to redress imbalances when coping with stress and facing challenges. Later, Helen Harris Perlman (1979) pointed out that the essence of what social workers do takes place in the interchange between ourselves and other people, and suggested that relationships have the potential to sustain us throughout life, affirming our sense of identity as well as a sense of oneness with others. These far-reaching therapeutic powers invested in the social work relationship discussed earlier in our history still holds true today.

Much of the literature continues to maintain that a healthy client–worker relationship infuses the helping process with energy and hope and becomes a medium through which to mobilize clients' strengths. Jeanne Marsh (2005) observes that "Social workers know that the connection between the worker and the client is the most powerful tool available to social workers, regardless of the treatment approach or modality they may be using" (p. 195). Relationships are the essence of our existence and continually influence and define who we are, how we feel, what we do, and the ways we live our lives.

According to Woods and Hollis (1990), the social work relationship can be a model for handling problems that arise with other people in our clients' lives. The client has the opportunity to identify with and incorporate the worker's personality and strengths in learning how to deal more effectively with difficult situations. While social work practitioners have always been concerned with the client–worker relationship, the focus has traditionally been on coping with problems. In the feminist relational approach, however, the emphasis shifts from merely coping, to growth and empowerment.

Most discussions of the professional relationship have revolved mainly around a description of essential worker characteristics that have been proven effective in establishing and sustaining a productive working relationship. Compton and her colleagues (2005) summarize these as follows. The social worker:

- evidences warmth;
- displays empathy;
- shows acceptance;
- is concerned;
- is genuine and congruent;
- shows commitment and obligation;
- uses authority and power appropriately.

Felix Biestek (1957) considered the relationship between worker and client to be "the channel of the entire casework process; through it flow the skills in intervention, study, diagnosis and treatment" (p. 4). He identified seven key features in the social work relationship reflecting professional values that promote growth and change and which continue to guide social work practice today: 1) individualization; 2) purposeful expression of feeling; 3) controlled emotional involvement; 4) acceptance; 5) non-judgmental attitude; 6) client self-determination; and 7) confidentiality. However, the curative powers of the therapeutic relationship described here are seen as separate and distinct elements, static attributes of a professional person, rather than dynamic interactional patterns between two people.

In contrast, the feminist relational approach places emphasis on the therapeutic milieu characterized by a sense of mutuality—a two-way interactive connection. It implicates the full range of emotions and thoughts that naturally flow between two or more persons. Thus, the client–worker dyad needs to be looked at as a behavioral system that functions in a reciprocal manner within a particular social and cultural milieu. This notion of mutuality is a key feature in the feminist relational approach and sets it apart from more traditional social work perspectives.

### Mutuality

Over the past decade, the Stone Center for Research and Clinical Studies has highlighted mutuality as a central component of a healthy relationship. The underlying assumption rests on the concept that mutual need and mutual aid are implicit in every society where interdependence ultimately leads to growth rather than isolation (Shulman, 2006). The notion of mutuality is implicit in the philosophy of a feminist relational approach and one that is often missing in the social work literature.

According to Stone Center pioneer Judith Jordan (1991c), the mutual exchange with a client is a setting in which "one is affecting the other and is being affected by the other; one extends oneself out to the other and is also receptive to the impact of the other" (p. 82). Simply stated, mutuality is the idea of reciprocity in relationship. Inherent in this approach is 1) an appreciation of the other as a unique, whole person; 2) an interest in and a cognitive awareness of the other's subjective state—who the other is, what he or she thinks and feels; 3) an ability to reveal one's own inner states to another; 4) a capacity to acknowledge one's own needs without manipulating the other; 5) a valuing of the process of enhancing the other's growth; and 6) a pattern of interaction in which both people are open to change.

Mutuality does not mean that each person in the relationship has equal power. Nor does mutuality imply an experience of sameness with the other. Appreciating differences while maintaining connection in a mutual exchange can be growth enhancing if there is sufficient respect, an understanding of the other's experience, an ongoing interest in their inner world, and the willingness to allow oneself to be affected by it (Jordan, 1991c). While the movement toward mutuality requires attunement to the clients' needs, it is not necessarily direct, immediate, or even continuous; it may be prone to fits and starts. The social worker can employ the following means in order to encourage the reciprocal impact of the worker and client system (Jordan, Kaplan, Miller, Stiver, & Surrey, 1997):

- disclose personal information;
- let the client know what you have learned from them;
- consider that the client has the most expertise on his or her problem;
- accept and validate the client's experiences, feelings, perceptions, thoughts, and their perceptions about you as a professional helper;
- express affection, care, and concern about the client.

First and foremost, the client–worker relationship is a partnership. In a non-dichotomous model, growth comes from the client's ability to become increasingly active within the relationship, eventually acting upon the environment with greater assertion (Kaplan, 1988). In many ways, technique is secondary to the worker's attitude embodied in these qualities:

- mutual respect;
- emotional availability;
- relational authenticity;
- relational awareness;
- responsiveness and presence;
- openness to influence.

The case of Linda, a 30-year-old, second generation Dominican young woman, illustrates the impact of mutuality on the client–worker relationship. Linda told me that she suffers from depression, and has always had a difficult time asserting herself with others. Subsequent to her divorce one year ago, she related that she was feeling isolated and lonely, and that it was hard for her to reach out to others. I had worked with Linda for about two months when she shared that she was having an affair with a married man at work. This relationship was basically the only gratifying one she had outside of her relationship with me. While Linda gave to others easily, she could not assert her own needs in return; hence, her relationships lacked mutuality.

Christmas and New Year were fast approaching and Linda was feeling particularly alone since her "boyfriend" would be with his wife. She dared not tell her parents or siblings about this relationship for fear of their judgment of her. They are religious, church-going people, who would view Linda's behavior as sinful. Her mother's strong tie to her Hispanic heritage and Linda's acculturation into the Anglo culture only widened the gap between them. Mom does not speak English nor does her world extend beyond where she lives and works. The literature indicates that close relationships between young Hispanic females and their mothers, when there is mutuality, understanding, and empathy, are factors that help young Latina women to negotiate the demands of both mainstream and Hispanic cultures. A close mother–daughter relationship has been correlated with higher levels of self-esteem and lower levels of depression (Genero, Miller, Surrey, and Baldwin, 1992). These findings are echoed in Linda's case.

I knew from previous sessions with Linda that when she becomes "down on herself," she retreats from others. I told Linda that her withdrawal and self-isolation scared me, given a previous suicide attempt she had made, and especially since the holidays are generally the worst times, even for the happiest of us. At the moment I said these words to her I felt Linda withdrawing from me.

In the past Linda had been teased and ridiculed by peers in school, her former mother-in-law, and her former husband. Repeated disconnections have been a part of Linda's life and she automatically avoids or retreats from others when she does not want to talk about something painful or when she feels uncomfortable. Linda lowered her head, became reticent, and moved her chair back. I felt disconnected from her and any attempt I made to empathize or reach out seemed useless. I said that I felt she was distancing herself from me as she does with others in her life. I reminded her that I cared about her, and I felt sad that she was feeling so alone—I wanted to help her, not hurt her.

Since Linda could not rely on her mother for a sense of connectedness, our relationship took on heightened significance. I let her know that I wanted to be there for her, and I felt frustrated and helpless that she had withdrawn emotionally. I imagined that she might also feel the same frustration and helplessness. I asked, "Do you want me to give up on you? Are you beginning to give up on yourself again?" I felt Linda's sense of hopelessness and told her I knew what it was like to feel alone. I let her know that in the past I too had withdrawn from others when I was in emotional pain, or when I felt "down on myself," and that those were the times when I needed other people the most. At those words, Linda started to cry. Her tears provided a way for her to express the painful well of emptiness that kept her so removed from others.

The reciprocal exchange that takes place in the client–worker relationship is made possible by the capacity of each participant for mutuality. As noted earlier, researchers have presented evidence that from birth, infants can express their intentions and needs to their caregiver, which results in a process of mutual regulation (Stern, 1985). Each member's actions are the complement of the partner; one person performs the action, the other receives it. The reciprocal flow of energy invested in the client–worker relationship sets the change process in motion. More recent research (Tronick & Weinberg, 1997) suggests that patterns of differentiation of self and other exist almost from birth:

> Exchanges with interactive partners which are well regulated generate positive affect, while mismatched exchanges produce negative affect. The expression of these affective states in turn communicates to the interactive partner to continue what he or she is doing or to change interactive behaviors.

(p. 56)

Mutuality rarely happens from the onset. Relationships evolve, change, and grow over time within multi-dimensional relational and cultural contexts. Helping clients connect with their full range of reactions, including the impact made on them by the social worker, enriches the dynamics of the interaction. Conversely, when social workers are able to connect with the impact clients have made on them, a truly relational experience is created.

In my relationship with Linda, I found it helpful to understand that because of past traumas and repeated disconnections, sometimes, those who yearn for connection the most hide parts of themselves from others, as well as from themselves. Miller and Stiver (1995) call this phenomenon the *paradox of connection*. The knowledgeable clinician, using mutually empathic skills, is aware of both sides of the dilemma: the desire on one side for secure attachment, and the fear of continued rejection or harm on the other. Children and adults alike use various strategies to either retreat into their private worlds or to act out aggressively to keep people away as a means of self-protection.

### Worker's Use of Self

The practice of feminist relational social work challenges professionals to critically reflect on the ways in which we use our selves in the helping relationship. The use of self is an ambiguous concept, and arguably one that has never been fully elaborated upon in the social work literature. Perhaps if we start by examining the use of self in the feminist relational approach we can better understand how social work can make use of this fundamental idea. In the relational feminist approach, the use of self is bound up with notions of mutuality, authenticity, boundaries, self-disclosure, dependency, transference and counter-transference issues, all of which are discussed in this chapter. Although these concepts overlap in practice, they are discussed separately for the purpose of clarification.

Although there may not be consensus on exactly what is meant by the use of self, clearly the worker's own unique self permeates his or her practice. Components of the worker's self include personality, culture, appearance, age, ethnicity, gender, and sexual orientation. Entering into another person's space requires sensitivity, knowledge, patience, compassion, skill, and keen self-awareness All these aspects of the self intersect and produce more than the sum of each part, encompassing a totally different and more elaborate cultural medium in which relational dynamics take place (Germain & Gitterman, 1996).

According to Jordan (1991c), in everyday life, "the other person is not there merely to take care of one's needs, to become a vessel for one's projections or transferences, or to be an object of discharge of instinctual impulses" (p. 82). By extension, when the client can see more than "just another social worker" in front of them, and can relate to the practitioner as a whole and separate individual, there is the potential for the client to become more invested in the helping process. If clients can then transfer this increased relational capacity to others in their lives, they become more effective in negotiating their environment and in forming healthier connections with others.

A brief example will illustrate this. After I had worked with Nina for three years, she missed a session and did not call. I phoned to see what had happened and left a message. She didn't call back until the following week. When we explored the meaning of her missed session, Nina herself connected her behavior with her tendency to avoid what she anticipated might be difficult; she wanted to terminate but did not know how to bring it up. I asked her how she thought I felt when she did not show or call. She said that she had no idea; she wasn't thinking of me. I let her know that I was worried and concerned about her, especially since Nina has had some serious health problems that led to hospitalization in the past.

Nina was moved by my concern, and added that when she was fearful of dealing with situations that made her anxious, she did not always consider others. She was able to acknowledge the fact that she avoided uncomfortable situations rather than assert herself, or confront the other person directly. This was a major issue in her marriage and in other relationships, especially with her mother. Knowing that I truly cared about her, and was not angry or disappointed as her mother and husband would have been if she stated her needs and wants, led to a deeper connection between us. Exploring this together made it possible for her to gain greater insight into herself, her relationship with others, and to experience behavioral patterns of which she was not aware.

In her relationship with her mother, Nina experienced the need to please her mother and make her proud. If she didn't satisfy her mother's needs and expectations, she was rejected by her, leaving her to feel a diminished sense of self. Nina realized that she avoided our session because she was afraid I would be hurt or displeased by her desire to terminate, and that then I would disconnect from her as her mother had always done. (In effect, she rejected me before she gave me the chance to reject her.) When I didn't react the way she had anticipated, she felt more validated and was more able to assert her needs.

The desire for self-assertion may engender tension when this need conflicts with girls' and women's need for security and acceptance. In her classic work, *Bonds of Love*, Jessica Benjamin (1988) concurs that tensions arise from people's need to differentiate themselves from others. Simultaneously, a fully formed self can only emerge from a supportive and close milieu, where one feels recognized and accepted. According to Benjamin, the tension between self-assertion and conformity constitutes opposite ends of a continuum, suspended in a delicate balance. Balancing both requires a paradigm shift—from an individualistic model of the self to one that allows uniqueness and difference to emerge within the context of connection. This balance is integral to what is called self-differentiation: the individual develops a self always aware of its distinctness while simultaneously needing to remain connected to others. In adolescence, this balance becomes even more precarious.

The following case example of my work with Leslie illustrates how as a social worker I used myself in a relationship with a 16-year-old female adolescent who was struggling to maintain the precarious balance between her need to develop her own sense of self, and her need to conform to the expectations of others.

When I initially met Leslie, she had been living with her father and brother in a suburb of a large metropolitan area for two years. She had lived in this same town with her parents until she was three and then the family decided to relocate to a small city in the Midwest. At the age of nine, Leslie's mother and father divorced and Dad moved back East. For the next five years, Leslie was shuffled back and forth between her mother and father. At age 15, she permanently moved in with her father.

Leslie's mother is an alcoholic who repeatedly goes on binges, which induce paranoid episodes for which she has been hospitalized on many occasions, leaving Leslie in charge of herself and her younger brother. After the parents separated, Leslie's father discovered that the children were living with a friend's family, so he petitioned for and received custody. He was also granted an Order of Protection from the court against Leslie's mother. At Leslie's request, her father contacted the community counseling center asking for help for his daughter.

During our first session, Leslie said, "I just wanted someone to talk to." Although she copes well with the many stressors that impact on her life, the identity crisis most teenagers face was exacerbated by her mixed ethnicity and family instability. Dad is Caucasian and Jewish and Mom is half-Caucasian, half Native American, and Catholic. Although her father is raising Leslie as Jewish, she identifies strongly with the Native American aspect of her heritage. Most of the time, Leslie feels disconnected from herself, her family, her heritage, her suburban community, her friends and family in the Midwest, and from her father, whom she frequently calls "an idiot." Until about age nine, Leslie recalls a warm and close relationship with her mother. Relying on her inherent strengths and early positive ties with her mother, she is quite resilient and mature, having had to grow up faster than many others her age. Her strongest connection is with her 13-year-old brother, for whom she often has had to play the role of surrogate parent.

I feel that my emotional presence is very important to Leslie. She needs someone on whom she can count to be there just for her—to understand how she feels and thinks, and to acknowledge her likes and dislikes. I ask her about her music and her taste in books. We have exchanged books and CDs. Surprisingly, we like some of the same things. Leslie has a strong need to be understood and to be "recognized" by others as she struggles to integrate a coherent self-identity.

In order for differentiation to evolve, Leslie needs to feel a secure attachment to another person, giving her a safe mooring to launch herself into the world. Her sophisticated cognitive skills and her insight help her to see her mother and father realistically, thereby reducing self-blame, guilt, and helplessness. Our connection is based on mutual respect, honesty, and authenticity: a contrast to the hypocrisy that she feels prevails in her life.

Although part of Leslie wants to conform to an image that will earn the approval of her peers, I continuously reinforce what is special and unique about her. Unlike the other girls in her town, she does not dress in the latest fashion, straighten her hair, nor does she paint her nails. She wears torn jeans, sneakers, and tee shirts most of the time. She likes poetry, plays the guitar, has eclectic taste in music, and likes to read the books of the "beat generation." In other words, she sees herself as "different," a unique individual who wants to be accepted for herself.

The need for relational resonance is great, especially for female adolescents. Girls have a strong need for connection, possibly because this is the stage in their lives where they are most likely to lose their "voice." There are many layers that become submerged, hidden away from others and even from the self. They begin to lose an authentic sense of connection because it is hard to find ways to show others who they really are (Gilligan, 1982). A good relationship with the mother, a pivotal figure during this stage, is still most important in helping the girl sort out the different, sometimes contrasting, aspects of herself. And a secure mother–daughter relationship is one of the most significant indicators of a healthy adolescence (Kaplan, Klein, & Gleason, 1985). My position as object replacement for Leslie's mother was reparative and may have helped to offset further damage (Miller & Stiver, 1997).

Since I generally agree with that aspect of feminist theory which emphasizes the importance of an adolescent girl maintaining a relationship with her mother, it was difficult for me to acknowledge that Leslie was not ready to reconnect with hers. The few times her mother telephoned, Leslie said that she "sounded drunk" and had not come through on promises she made. Leslie wasn't ready to see her mother and knew she had to protect herself from further disappointment. I shared with Leslie that I fully supported and respected her decision—in many ways she seemed more mature than her mother, which I knew contributed to her feeling of being cut off from that most significant relationship, resulting in her inner sense of isolation and loneliness.

A willingness to bring observations out into the open and to elicit client feedback can provide clients with vital information about themselves and their interactions with other social systems. This is best accomplished if the worker is able to tolerate, work with, and sustain tension in the relationship. The fact that people are so complex makes it hard to predict the outcome of any helping relationship. Energy flows in many directions as long as interpersonal boundaries are permeable. The normal tension that exists in the client–worker relational system is influenced by, but not limited to the following: 1) our degree of authenticity; 2) how we regulate closeness and distance between ourselves and clients; 3) our ability to sustain connection in spite of disruption and conflict; and 4) what we do or do not disclose.

## Self-Disclosure

The notion of self-disclosure is related to the use of self and the concept of mutuality. Workers who adopt a more feminist relational approach agree that the more the worker shares, the more connected some clients may feel with the worker, and the more productive the relationship can be. However, according to Cooper and Lesser (2002), this "ethic of mutuality" in the therapeutic relationship does not *mandate* self-disclosure. The more traditional, psychoanalytic perspective is that worker self-disclosure is merely an attempt to gratify the client and therefore is deemed an obstacle in the therapeutic process (Raines, 1996). While this view has prevailed in some circles, as social work theory embraced systemic, ego-oriented, and interactional models, social workers themselves began to realize that there is no such thing as complete neutrality. Thus self-disclosure has received more attention and has gained wider acceptance, particularly in the feminist relational model. In general, clinicians using a feminist model of relational theory might be more inclined to reveal parts of their authentic selves in order to connect with the client (Dewane, 2006).

The parameters of what the worker shares as opposed to what a friend, a work associate, or a family member shares are, naturally, different. Of course, selectivity is key. Be clear about what you're revealing, the reasons you're revealing it, and make it consistent with your understanding of who your client is and what they need from you. Timing is also critical. Since workers help clients mediate reality, their reactions often provide helpful feedback. Focusing on the "here and now" in the relationship can provide "in-vivo" learning that facilitates growth and allows the client to gain a fuller recognition of how they impact others.

Sensitivity is paramount in trying to gauge how much the client can actually "hear" of the worker's negative feelings, such as disappointment or anger. More positive feelings, such as wanting to protect or care for the client, may be rejected as well, since those can be too threatening if the client has a need to maintain more formal boundaries or to reject help altogether (Miller & Stiver, 1991). Disclosure, therefore, must be based on an accurate assessment of clients and their present state of mind. Clearly, if the client is feeling overwhelmed, overstressed, or too vulnerable, it is best to focus exclusively on him or her.

Disclosure is a tricky thing to negotiate. There is the fear that you may share too much, but there is also the danger of sharing too little. Balance is key. Keep your client's needs in the forefront. Disclosure of the worker's experience is fine but *only* if it serves your client—not you. Janet Surrey

(1991) suggests that not disclosing anything may have a negative effect on those clients who are prone to isolation or who have poor social skills. They may interpret this as their own failure to relate effectively or they may feel that the worker is not interested in them, resulting in a disconnection. However, the worker should not feel compelled to immediately respond to a client's request for personal information.

For example, if a client asks me if I have any children, or if I am married, or what my sexual orientation or religion is, I may answer and then explore the meaning this has for them. Sometimes I will explore the reason for their question and then choose whether or not to respond. Many times those kinds of questions are related to concerns about their own lives, or whether I can understand them and their situation, or whether there is common ground to build a relationship on. It may be very helpful, for example, for a client who is going through a divorce to know that their worker has been divorced as well. The worker can convey whatever their experience was with the intent to facilitate identification without sharing too many of the details, possibly reducing any sense of shame the client may have in the process.

If a worker discloses how she handled a particular situation, clients can feel intimidated or embarrassed, thinking that they do not have the skills to do it that way. Clients need reminding that everyone is unique and that individuals handle things differently. Disclosure must be done in a manner that helps clients learn and grow, without making them feel that they must do it *your* way. The important thing is to encourage clients to try out new behaviors compatible with who they are or who they want to be.

Then there are some clients who do not want to know anything about you. They refrain from asking any questions and seem more comfortable keeping the relationship more formal. As a general rule, social workers should avoid divulging any material that 1) they themselves have not worked through, 2) sounds like a confession, which may make clients feel they have to protect or reassure the worker, 3) is not relevant to the helping relationship, the agency function, or that the client does not seem interested in, 4) is beyond the worker's comfort zone, and 5) is beyond the client's comfort zone.

It is important that the worker respect the client's boundaries and maintain acute sensitivity in terms of what is safe to disclose—just as in a marriage, the optimal emotional distance between two people is mutually regulated. The decision to disclose any personal information to the client is based on the assumption that the worker is able to focus on the client's needs and wants without using the client–worker situation to gratify his or her own needs. I strongly believe that the ability to exert this kind of judgment is closely related to the worker's level of maturity and self-awareness.

The case of Tracy illustrates the conscious use of self-disclosure in a manner that enhanced the client–worker relationship. Tracy is a Caucasian single mother of Justin, an 18-year-old biracial male. Her relationship with her son is a major source of pain, anger, and disappointment to Tracy. According to her they were once close, but now communication has totally broken down. She and Justin's father divorced when he was four, and Justin has not seen his dad since he was eight. At that time, the father was arrested for possession of drugs and fired from his job as a detective in the police force. Neither Tracy nor Justin ever talked about the circumstances surrounding his dad's disappearance, nor do they talk about him now. He remains the "elephant in the room." The secrecy about Justin's father has had destructive effects on everyone. As a young man trying to establish an identity in a racist world, not knowing anything about his father and his father's family is a denial of Justin's heritage and his sense of reality.

For the last two years, Justin has been using alcohol and marijuana and dealing cocaine. Most recently he was arrested for possession of marijuana. It appears that Justin harbors a deep need for an attachment with his biological father, demonstrated by the fact that his behavior replicates the older man's. According to Miller & Stiver (1995), individuals like Justin often become fearful of becoming close to others because of past neglect, humiliation, and loss. In response, they begin to isolate parts of themselves, and develop a repertoire of strategies that keep others at a distance—safe enough from being hurt again.

According to Tracy, Justin is opposed to any request she makes of him, even one as small as having dinner together on Sunday evenings. She feels he is "just a boarder" in the house. The reality of raising a difficult adolescent is overwhelming to her. The sense of helplessness she feels is contrary to her usual self-image of a competent woman in control of her life. What Tracy perceives as a loss of power or failure in her maternal role she has turned against herself. She has not gone out socially in years, has not invested in her community, nor has she done much of anything to feel good about herself.

Although she presents as a stoic, independent woman, Tracy actually feels hurt, unloved, lonely, and frustrated. She has few social connections or supports. Tracy has invested her whole life in Justin, and feels a deep sense of shame in believing she has failed as a parent. This has caused her to further isolate herself from friends and family.

Taking on the responsibility to meet the needs of others begins at birth, often leading women to become more "other-focused." The implications of this are two-fold: 1) women have been trained to look to others for affirmation and value, placing them in a vulnerable position; and 2) women have been given the message by society that self-denial is characteristic of good mothering. Yet if one ignores one's own needs, the anger connected to depriving the self may accumulate and initiate a cycle of inadequate mothering and low self-esteem for both mother and child. Both Tracy and Justin were caught in this cycle.

I thought about my own adolescence—how I had rebelled against my parents in an effort to establish a clearer sense of self. I shared this with Tracy, which led us to talk about the ways in which she rebelled against her parents during adolescence. Through this discussion, I was hoping that she could gain a greater degree of empathy for her son. Although Tracy desperately wanted a closer relationship with Justin, she was not able to see how her anger pushed him away. Without realizing it, she was creating a situation in which she disconnected from Justin, he then disconnected from her, and both experienced a vicious cycle of rejection.

Tracy and I talked about her disappointment and pain. I commented that if she and Justin were to have any relationship at all, approaching him in an angry manner would only further humiliate and alienate him. I suggested that it may be best to use her own feelings of hurt and disappointment to let him know how much she wanted to be a part of his life, rather than give in to the impulse to cut herself off or react out of anger. I shared my experience with my own adolescent children; that when I was vulnerable and open, they responded in kind. Also, no matter how angry or hurt I was, I always tried to remember that I was the grown-up and had to make the first move when communication broke down. I let her know how hard this could be for me at times. (This brought up memories of my relationship with my own mother—a relationship in which we would go for weeks without speaking until I approached her. I consciously chose not to disclose this as I did not think it relevant, although it did make me more sensitive to Tracy's pain.)

I did relate to Tracy that it was hard for me at times and maybe for her too, to be the "adult" with our teenage children. I said, "When we are hurt or feel rejected, our impulse is to lash out and hurt back, but that just creates more obstacles." Communicating with Tracy in this more personal way modeled how she could be more open with Justin to engage in a freer give and take. I conveyed my belief that if she could reveal more about herself— her thoughts, her disappointments, her experiences—to her son, she would come across as more approachable and accessible. In turn, Justin might respond more openly to her.

As our relationship grew over time, Tracy gradually made significant changes, which in turn, had an impact on Justin. For example, with my support Tracy began to connect with others, which helped reduce her isolation. I encouraged her to talk with her sister-in-law who was in recovery. She understood Tracy's situation and could offer the support she needed. Tracy's two brothers also got involved, so Justin now had two adult male figures to partially compensate for the absence of his father. Tracy then joined a parent self-help support group, and, to her surprise, connected with many of the other group members. The relationships with her family and with members of the group helped her to feel more secure and to set more consistent limits for Justin.

As Tracy became closer with members of her parents' group, she created the opportunity to share similar experiences in an atmosphere of mutuality. She was able to give to others and get back in return. This was rewarding for Tracy, and she began to seek out more connections and felt part of a larger community. She became a volunteer at the city performing arts center and was thinking of working in a local political campaign. Now that she was meeting people, was more connected to her own community, and had more of her own life, she could relax her hold on Justin. Reciprocally, Justin began to feel that he could more comfortably move away from his mom, while at the same time maintain a new and different relationship with her.

### Relational Authenticity

What is meant by relational authenticity? Working in a relational way and using the authentic self implies that the worker participates in a relationship in which he or she feels comfortable enough in the presence of the other to be "real." Thus, the practitioner's verbalizations and actions will hopefully be congruent and conducive to engaging the client in a relationship that facilitates trust and growth (Miller et al., 1999).

According to Jean Baker Miller and colleagues (1999), the worker's disclosure of true feelings, selective sharing of experiences, lack of defensiveness, and presentation of a less-than-perfect authority promotes a sense of relational authenticity that can be the impetus for a real exchange. Instead of stressing the importance of neutrality, the client–worker relationship is more productive when the worker is authentically present and participating in the relationship with the client as an equal or "near equal" partner.

The following example illustrates the importance of the worker's ability to remain open to differences of all kinds—cultural, class, gender, sexual orientation, and value systems. Nancy is a 35-year-old, second generation Latina woman. She is highly intelligent and successful in her career. Her competence in the workplace enabled her to get a raise and a promotion within a relatively short period of time. Her fiancé Tony, a 45-year-old, second generation Italian, is much more traditional, and expects his wife-to-be to assume the same roles and responsibilities in their home as his mother had. Although Nancy was willing to go along with this to a point, she expressed her doubts about their long-term compatibility. She was willing to do a good deal of the domestic tasks but didn't want this to undermine her career.

Nancy knew that being a more traditional housewife like Tony's mom wouldn't quite fit her, but she really wanted to marry. She was emotionally dependent on Tony, loved him, and believed she could be happy with him. She asked me what I thought. I stated that different household arrangements work best for different couples; the reality of her experience is that she might have to compromise her ideals of gender equality if she wanted to have a successful relationship. (Hochschild and Machung (2003) document that even when women have demanding careers they end up doing more of the household chores than men.)

I told Nancy that, like many women, I too have struggled with dependency needs. Being authentic involves being true to your values and ideals without judging another. I thought that it was important to help Nancy examine her own feelings about gender roles and whether she would be comfortable adjusting it to fit her desire for security and a successful marriage. At the same time, I was honest that it would be hard to me to compromise my career to assume a greater share of the household responsibilities than my partner. However, I let Nancy know that I thought it was very important that she make a decision that best fit her needs and wishes and those of her fiancé. I wondered aloud if she thought there was room for negotiation and compromise. I believed that my role was to help her clarify the extent to which she was willing to accommodate difference or negotiate conflict without losing self-esteem or a sense of control over her life.

This notion of authenticity has many implications for the way the worker uses himself or herself in the relationship. When we are fully present with the client, we can move with greater ease. When we are in touch with our own feelings, thoughts, and intuitions—our true selves—we are moving toward becoming more integrated, more authentic workers; something which continues as we mature into our professional roles through training, supervision, and commitment to our own growth. The feminist relational notion of authenticity is congruent with many of the basic notions presented in the social work literature. Hepworth et al. (2006) define it as "the sharing of the self by relating in a natural, sincere, spontaneous, open, and genuine manner" (p. 107). Being authentic or genuine involves relating personally to the other so that expressions are spontaneous rather than contrived. Although the worker can be naturally spontaneous, both perception and judgment are always modified by professional training. It is important to remember that spontaneity is not the same as being impulsive, the latter being more of an unpredictable response without regard for consequences. Spontaneity, rather, is an unguarded, unconstrained, unforced, and unaffected response. Direct and spontaneous articulation of the worker's feelings is acceptable as long as it is not based on the worker's own needs, but rather guided by therapeutic intention.

As social workers, we are trained to use ourselves in an egalitarian way, which means that we are keenly aware of redistributing as much of the power in the relationship as possible, given the parameters of our role. Regardless of setting, the feminist relational approach dictates that one is, above all, honest and open about purpose, goals, and possible outcomes of the helping process, thereby maximizing the principle of self-determination. Sometimes the worker will make an error, a poorly timed intervention perhaps, resulting in the client disconnecting. Whatever the precipitating factor, mistakes are inevitable. It is the willingness and responsibility of the worker to at least explore what happened and attempt to repair any damage that are most important. The goal is to move from disconnection to connection without the client disengaging from or disrupting the relationship. In essence, the social worker must be willing to learn from the client and be able to admit when he or she has made a mistake.

*The Role of Transference–Counter-Transference in the*
*Relational Model*

In the 1950s and 1960s, Helen Harris Perlman (1957) and Florence Hollis (1964) cautioned social workers to maintain firm boundaries in the service of controlling transference and counter-transference reactions, thinking that expression of these could distort the relationship. Now that we have moved toward using ourselves in a more open way, the way in which we understand transference phenomena needs to be reframed. Originally associated with Freudian theory, these terms refer to the transfer of unresolved feelings about significant figures onto the other person in the relationship. When viewed in a relational context, transference phenomena is part of a normative, therapeutic process. It is not unusual that a social worker in a helping role would remind the client of someone who has been significant in his or her life. It becomes the worker's responsibility to guide the client in exploring, understanding, and "giving voice" to these feelings and thoughts. Many times the mysterious notion of "transference" is accessible to consciousness and can be used for increased insight about how we relate to other people.

Miller and Stiver (1997) ask us to distinguish which of those reactions are more anchored in the past, and which are more reflective of the present relationship between worker and client. Sometimes this is difficult to determine since, realistically, things are not purely one or the other, but a mixture of both. The more self-aware one strives to be, the better chance one has at distinguishing the two. Sometimes it is helpful to discuss memories of one's past relationships in a context of safety, particularly if these memories evoke strong feelings such as anger, fear, or love. We all elicit feelings in each other, and it is important not to negate those, but rather to process them so clients can learn how to deal with their feelings in constructive ways (Wishnie, 2005). By working in the transference, the client can be helped to gain a greater understanding of past relationships in which distortions and misunderstandings have led to disconnection.

The relational view of countertransference includes anything that helps or hurts a therapist's ability to maintain a real connection with a client—to be truly present and truly aware. Rather than see it as an impediment, countertransference can be an opportunity for the social worker to learn more about the client by examining all the thoughts and feelings stirred up in the interaction (Miller & Stiver, 1991; Miller & Stiver, 1997). Much of the time the practitioner is picking up on feelings the client is experiencing and cannot acknowledge. Once aware of these dynamics, he or she can be more empathic and responsive to the client's distress.

The following case illustrates the worker's ability to balance acceptance of the client and an understanding of the transference while setting limits on unacceptable behavior. I had been seeing Michael, a white, 34-year-old man, for about six months. Upon returning from the bathroom during one session, Michael's zipper was open and his penis was exposed. I felt uncomfortable but decided it was important to comment on this and said, "I don't know if you are aware, but you didn't close your zipper when you re-entered the office." Michael said he was sorry and got up to do so. I asked how he felt when I confronted him because he looked ruffled. He disclosed that he purposely did this and had been exposing himself to women for years. He liked to take them "by surprise" and got a thrill out of embarrassing them. The irony is that Michael suffered from shame his whole life due to an over controlling, critical mother. His father in turn was verbally demeaning and abusive to his mother. He didn't understand why she couldn't stand up to him. His anger at women came out in the only way he felt he could control them—to scare and shame them as *he* had been. I was another female authority figure who he feared could shame him like his mother had. Perhaps his behavior was a way of expressing his anger at me for having more power than he had.

I did not feel angry or uncomfortable once I brought his behavior patterns to his attention. In fact, I felt relieved. I believe Michael was also relieved that his secret was revealed. I shared with Michael that I appreciated his honesty, and was glad he was willing to work on his issues with me. But he needed clear boundaries and limit setting and I let him know that I would not tolerate any acting out.

### Boundaries

According to Judith Jordan, boundaries are often depicted in traditional literature as a means of protection rather than as potential avenues of exchange. The boundaried self is restricted in openness and emotional responsiveness (Jordan, 1984). A frequent criticism of feminist-oriented relational theories involves the notion of boundaries. Traditional approaches hold that a clear separation between worker and client maintains professionalism and averts over-involvement. I prefer to see boundaries as established by continuous and natural interaction. On one hand, the participants have some need to make contact with each other, on the other hand they also have a need to protect themselves and maintain distance. As trust is built, natural boundaries are established from working together and sharing intimate moments.

Compton et al. (2005) use the term *boundary* to identify the places where one system or subsystem ends and the other begins. Kirst-Ashman and Hull (1995) describe boundaries as "invisible barriers which surround individuals and subsystems, regulating the amount of contact with others" (p. 317).

What distinguishes the relational approach from other models is the belief that boundaries can represent a place of meeting rather than a line of demarcation (Jordan & Dooley, 2000). The relational perspective stresses that because individuals thrive when they engage in growth-fostering relationships, client–worker boundaries need to be flexible to allow for the flow of reciprocal energy that empowers and encourages client participation (Jordan, 1991d).

Contrary to a more traditional psychodyanamic approach in which there is overt concern about maintaining emotional distance, the relational social worker allows for a wide range of feelings and thoughts in the moment, facilitating a sense of connection (Jordan, 1984). However, feeling deeply with the other is not the same thing as "merger," nor does it suggest a "blurring of the self with the other," as some male theorists have suggested. Although boundaries may be regulated by both client and worker depending on the setting, the reality is that workers can set limits based on their assessment of the client and his or her needs. Clearly, boundaries are helpful in providing safety. But flexibility and permeability allow the worker to emphasize and respect the vulnerability of the other.

At times, there might even be a sense of fusion between client and worker, although this does not necessarily mean a loss of boundaries. According to Berzoff (1989), females found to be at the highest levels of ego development described the phenomenon of fusion in their closest friendships. This indicates a deep ability for closeness, but at the same time, a clear sense of self in relation to the other. Perhaps a state of *interdependence* would be ideal, one in which healthy dependency needs are accepted, fluid, shared, and mutually met, while each person maintains a strong sense of self in a relational context of trust and intimacy.

### Dependency

The degree of dependency that the worker fosters is related to the worker's assessment of the client-in-their-situation. Some clients require a greater degree of dependency than others, for example, the frail elderly, those in crisis, and children. Inherent in all of us is a striving toward autonomy, and the push toward growth usually supersedes the wish to remain helpless. Negotiating the tension between dependence and independence is necessary and is to be respected, not faulted. The worker's emotional and physical availability (similar to those of a parent) can provide a corrective emotional experience. As the individual matures, dependency needs remain part of every relationship in some form. Sometimes the worker has to help the client learn to be dependent on them while working incrementally toward increasing autonomy, especially when the client needs emotional and physical replenishment in preparation for more independent functioning down the road.

Irene Stiver (1991) defines dependency as "a process counting on other people to provide help in coping, physically and emotionally, with the experiences and tasks encountered in the world when one has not sufficient skill, confidence, energy, and/or time" (p. 160). Her definition stresses dependency not as a static condition, but rather one that changes along with opportunities and circumstances, making an ongoing assessment all the more important.

Dependency has to do with relying on something or someone else for support, and is not a condition that is held in high esteem in our individualistic "bootstraps" culture. Yet for some clients whose basic needs were not met early on, it may be absolutely essential to encourage dependency. In fact, it is impossible to become independent without first having been dependent to a certain degree. Dependency is not a value-free concept. In our individualistic society that extols self-reliance, the word carries pejorative connotations of weakness, vulnerability, helplessness. Whereas the male-constructed ethic of self-reliance, independence, and individualism has permeated our cultural ideas, men and women are encouraged to discard or conceal rather than acknowledge feelings of dependency, or the need for attachment, caring, and support. These attitudes have trickled down to the social work profession, which often results in a bias against those clients who are more dependent than others.

In the process of forming relationships, dependency is often labeled as an expression of regressive needs (Miller, 1976). However, in the feminist relational approach, dependency is not seen as inherently regressive, nor does being dependent necessarily equal losing the ability to cope. Women's affiliative needs do not preclude their ability to maintain a consolidated identity, nor do men's independent maneuvers preclude their need for connection. To compensate for cultural bias, the worker must respect the dependency needs of all clients and accept and regard these non-judgmentally.

Feminist thinkers, such as Carol Gilligan (1982), have noted a cultural bias against permitting and encouraging dependence. Gilligan discusses the differences in how dependency issues are experienced by women and men. Women have more social pressure to disown their dependency needs. As a consequence, they often keep their distance from others to avoid being "reeled in." The fact that men have more difficulties in acknowledging their vulnerability and their need for others has caught the attention of several other theorists. Dorothy Dinnerstein (1997) takes the position that a man's effort to achieve a sexual identity different from his mother propels him to repudiate levels of autonomous functioning.

## Social Work Best Practices for Building the Client–Worker Relationship

As a social worker you can strengthen the client–worker relationship through practicing a number of proven techniques.

- The client–worker relationship serves as a model for other relationships. The social worker has the opportunity to use the relationship as a restorative experience for the client.
- The social worker must be genuine and congruent at all times, expressing commitment and a sense of caring on a consistent basis.

- Mutuality is critical to the client–worker relationship. The social work clinician must facilitate a reciprocal exchange of feelings and thoughts between worker and client.
- The social work clinician focuses on significant disconnections as well as connections in the client's life space; especially, those relationships which impede or enhance the client's ability to feel empowered.
- The desire and yearning for relational ties with others is strong throughout the life cycle and impacts the way clients deal with stress, trauma, and normative phases of human growth and development. The social worker seeks to mobilize positive relational networks, relational ties and exchanges in the environment to enhance clients' coping capacities.

In summary, the mutual exchange that occurs between the client system and worker is made possible by the capacity of each participant for mutuality, mutual respect, emotional availability, relational responsiveness and awareness, openness to being moved by the other, and mutual empathy. In the next chapter we will explore the notion of mutual empathy as a particularly significant relational aspect of the social work relationship.

# 4 Relational Theory and Empathy

## A Feminist Perspective

For thousands of years, people have been aware of what is now commonly referred to as *empathy*. In ancient Greece, philosophers expressed their understanding with the word *empatheia*, which implies an active appreciation of another person's feeling experience (Astin, 1967). The English word derives from the German *Einfühlung*, which literally means "feeling oneself into." Empathy was introduced into our clinical vocabulary by German psychologist Edward Tichener at the turn of the twentieth century and was generally accepted as the equivalent of *Einfühlung* (Berger, 1987). Almost every modern conceptualization of the word shares the notion that empathy involves the capacity to participate in the inner experience of another or to comprehend the feelings or ideas of another.

Throughout the twentieth century, social workers have been influenced by Freudian and ego-oriented theorists in their understanding and application of empathy. Freud conceived of empathy as a cognitive technique that enhanced the therapist's ability to enter into the internal world of the client, thereby facilitating accurate interpretation of unconscious material (Bohart & Greenberg, 1997). By exploring the patient's thoughts and feelings without judging them, the use of empathy could help the therapist gain insight into the patient's motivation. Despite Freud's use of empathy as an intrapsychic process, he generally regarded it as a background variable with limited curative powers.

In more classical psychoanalytic thinking, the therapist is expected to suppress any and all feelings evoked by the patient in order to avoid countertransference (Basch, 1988). It was thought that communicating emotionality might distort the neutrality of the relationship and impede the development of the transference. So it was considered best that the clinician remain a passive listener and convey a neutral, objective stance (Bohart et al., 1997).

Some psychoanalytically minded theorists consider empathy, along with subjectivity, suspended rationality, and emotionality, to be distinctly feminine traits. A parallel has been made between a worker's empathy for a client and a mother's empathy for her child, reaffirming a tie to the female role, one often devalued in our society (Berger, 1987). When social work incorporated modern psychodynamic theories into its knowledge base from the 1950s through the 1970s—ego psychology, client-centered theory, self-psychology, and object relations theory—the emphasis shifted from drive theory to the role of the relational milieu in producing and reproducing healthy growth and development. It was during this time that empathy came to play a more central role in social work practice.

## Relational Contexts: Psychological Metaphors for Empathy

Object-relations theorist D.W. Winnicott (1965) considered empathy and emotional attunement to be *the* most crucial elements in mothering, which suggests a parallel between the "good enough" mother and the "good enough" social worker. According to Winnicott, the mother's anticipation of her baby's needs and the proper timing in meeting those needs are the basis for the development of a healthy, creative self. Similarly, through the use of empathy, the worker provides a facilitating environment for growth, development, and the enhancement of adaptive skills. If, in the safety of the environment, the client experiences the worker as empathic and accepting, it is more likely that an authentic self will unfold, setting the stage for a more trusting relationship with the worker (Greenberg et al., 1983).

Fox (2001) calls this protective therapeutic milieu the "safe house," a place where the social worker supplies some of the nurturance missing from the client's earlier experience. Through the use of empathy, the social worker's task is to enable clients to feel understood and accepted enough to risk revealing hidden parts of themselves. Simultaneously, the worker relaxes his/her own boundaries, so that the reaction clients evoke in the clinician become more readily accessible. It is this kind of relational "holding" that maximizes the therapeutic value of empathy and has the potential for far-reaching interpersonal change.

Carl Rogers (1951), the father of client-centered therapy, identified empathy as "the ability to perceive the internal frame of reference of another with accuracy without ever losing the 'as if' condition" (p. 210). According to Rogers, empathy is not only used as a means to an end, but also as an end in itself, and involves a focus on understanding the subtleties of the client's experience in the moment. It is the clinician's attempts to reflect understanding of the client's world that remain at the core of the healing process.

Kohut (1977) views the capacity to empathize as a cornerstone of the development of an integrated sense of self. His school of self-psychology stresses the primacy of the worker's ability to understand, and then reflect on, the client's subjective experience. Kohut defines empathy as "the capacity to experience the patient's inner life while remaining objective" (p. 16). "Mirroring" the client's reality—feelings, thoughts, experiences, and perceptions—helps build a cohesive sense of self (Greenberg et al., 1983). Thus, empathic responses on the part of the clinician can create a milieu that potentially compensates for repeated empathic failures in childhood; those moments when the caretaker did not tune in and respond in an accurate and timely manner to the child's wants and needs (Eisenberg & Strayer, 1987).

## Contemporary Definitions and Characteristics

Many social work theorists consider empathy as central to human experience and a critical element in professional practice (Hepworth et al., 2006; Germain et al., 1996; Raines, 1990). Keefe (1976) defines it as a "set of behaviors that constitute a skill central to effective social work intervention at every level" (p. 10). It has also been referred to as "the ability of the practitioner to understand, as accurately as possible, what it is that a client is experiencing from the client's frame of reference" (Boyle et al., 2006, p. 113). Although social work scholars conceptualize empathy a bit differently, all highlight the same essential elements:

- active listening;
- genuineness and positive regard;
- a sense of understanding;
- accurate attunement to emotional and cognitive processes.

Most social workers recognize that without empathy, there would be fewer engaged clients and fewer successful outcomes. Studies consistently identify empathy as one of the critical variables affecting the helping process and closely correlated with effective outcomes in social work practice. For example, Truax and Mitchell (1971) found a direct correlation between the therapist's empathy, warmth, and genuineness, and client change. Shulman (2006) corroborates these findings, citing empathy as a powerful ingredient in building a constructive working relationship.

## Conveying Empathy

For most social workers, empathy involves not only the ability to enter into the experience of another, but also the ability to communicate that understanding and create an atmosphere of validation and support. Once demonstrated, the client may be more likely to trust that the clinician is there to help and, as a result, may work harder and more collaboratively.

Although Woods et al. (1999) view empathy as an essential element in demonstrating a sense of caring for the client and enhancing his or her feeling of being understood and respected, they recommend at the same time that workers contain their own feelings. Their position is that if workers do not harness their own personal responses, those responses could potentially interfere with the client's own process and ultimately circumvent transference reactions.

In standard social work practice, empathy is generally used descriptively and in conjunction with other basic skills, such as reflection and clarification—with the caveat that the social worker should not focus too intensely on the client's affective state nor take on the emotions experienced by the client as if they were the clinician's own. According to Hepworth and his colleagues (2006), the first dimension of clinical practice, *recognition*, involves mainly insight and cognition; the second, *demonstration*, is a comprehension of the client's inner experience through accurate reflection of thoughts and feelings.

While empathic communication involves "stepping *into* the shoes" of the other, Hepworth et al. argue that the clinician must simultaneously remain *outside* of the client's inner emotional world "to avoid being overwhelmed by his or her fears, angers, joys, and hurts" (2006, p. 87). Accordingly, these authors do not believe the worker should focus too intensely on the client's affective state, or take on the emotions experienced by the client as if those were the worker's own, since it might result in the worker losing his/her own perspective, thus reducing the ability to be helpful.

Much of traditional literature suggests that social workers should never abandon neutrality (Keefe, 1976; Raines, 1990). This idea implies that retaining separateness is a critically important dimension in the helping process. According to Keith-Lucas:

> Empathy is the worker's understanding of the feelings the other has about the situation, knowing inside oneself how uncomfortable and desperate these feelings may be for the client, but never claiming these feelings for oneself as the helping person.
>
> (1976, pp. 80–81)

Compton et al. (2005) best capture what social workers see as its inherent tensions and contradictions: "Empathy requires what may seem to many beginning workers to be antithetical qualities—the capacity to feel emotion deeply and yet to remain separate enough from it to be able to use [that] knowledge" (p. 151).

Social workers who embrace a more traditional psychoanalytic view, often err on the side of maintaining too much distance, thereby making it difficult to fully engage in a satisfying relationship: one in which the client is able to trust that the worker is genuinely "there." Modern-day workers are cautioned to maintain clear and separate boundaries so as to avoid the possibility of over-identifying with the client. It is here that the relational/ cultural model and mainstream social work approach to empathy part ways.

One of the basic differences between traditional social work practice and the feminist approach is the degree to which the practitioner remains "outside" the client's experience. Keen self-awareness and the ability to maintain clear yet flexible boundaries are the most important ingredients in being able to resonate deeply with the feelings and experiences of the client while remaining closely connected to one's own feelings and experiences.

While traditional concepts of empathy call for the worker to understand the client and to express that understanding, feminist relational theorists conceptualize this phenomenon more broadly, as a reciprocal, dynamic process, embedded in the client–worker relational/cultural context, growing and changing over time. The worker, who expresses empathy in the form of interest in and concern for the other, serves as a role model in helping clients learn ways to enhance all of their relationships—with family, with friends, and with members of their communities. Similar to Rogers' (1951) ideas, feminist relational theorists believe that empathy provides a secure and safe context that validates and reaffirms the client's sense of self. Thus, empathy in the therapeutic process increases the client's ability to feel free to be his/her "true self" in the presence of another (Stiver & Miller, 1988).

## The Intersubjective Approach

Jessica Benjamin (1988) offers a relational model that considers empathy from an intersubjective point of view; that is, the client and worker recognizing each other's subjective states from their separate vantage points. The notion of *intersubjectivity* implies a high level of emotional attunement and sharing, and can serve as an instrument of therapeutic change. Both client and clinician recognize that they have an impact on the other, are intent on learning more about themselves and the other, and hopefully grow from the experience. According to Benjamin, through the empathic, confirming response of the therapist, the client comes to feel recognized, affirmed, and valued.

This recognition implies that the worker and the client have entered into each other's emotional world, thereby reducing the distance between them. The worker is not seen as merely an object of the client's needs, but rather as a separate entity, whose empathic responsiveness allows the client to feel more "real." The idea of being recognized as a person in one's own right, and not just as an extension of another's hopes, wants, beliefs, and needs, can be empowering for the client. The energy released in this mutual recognition has the potential to nourish the client's desire to explore and develop other relationships.

## Lara's Case: Empathy in Action

Lara, a 27-year-old Albanian woman, had seen many social workers before coming to the community mental health center where I practiced. During her adolescence Lara suffered from major depression and was hospitalized after a suicide attempt. She had low self-esteem, few friends, and tended to isolate. Not only did Lara think little of herself, but she felt that others did not care about her, either. She considered herself unattractive and believed she had nothing of interest to offer anyone. Having come to the United States from Albania at age six, Lara entered school unfamiliar with the English language. Consequently, she had difficulty reading and was placed in a special education class.

During her adolescence Lara was overweight and was teased by her peers. She usually avoided people because she felt "stupid" and did not know what to say. I felt the pain of Lara's isolation and shame, and let her know that her sense of worthlessness and continuous rejection of herself made me feel sad.

From the painful life experiences and feelings Lara shared with me I understood why she felt uncomfortable with others. However, I experienced her very differently than she experienced herself. I said, "You come across to me as a caring person who gives a lot of herself to others. I believe that people would appreciate your sincerity and kindness as much as I do when they get to know you better." I wanted Lara to see herself in a different and more realistic light and to feel the positive impact she had made on me. It was important for Lara to know that she mattered to me, particularly since she had felt so excluded and humiliated for so much of her childhood and young adult years. The experience of "mattering," of having an impact on the other person, increases one's sense of relational competence. Lara became tearful and said that my understanding and caring meant a great deal to her.

Lara's story led me to re-live some of my own adolescent memories of feeling lonely, which made it even easier for me to feel her pain. I too felt out of place when I entered a very large urban high school much younger than most of the other students. Being new to the neighborhood, I knew very few students in the school. Although I did not share Lara's exact experiences, I could put myself in her place and authentically feel with her. My ability to resonate with her on a deep level helped us to create a mutually empathic connection together. Being able to feel previously walled-off pain, and to form a different relational image of herself based on our mutual interaction and the empathy we shared, Lara began feel more comfortable with herself and others. She slowly reached out to old friends and current acquaintances in an attempt to make new connections and reduce her self-imposed isolation.

A core feature of Benjamin's (1998) framework is the notion that any similarity between two people coexists in an uneasy balance with their inherent differences—cultural, psychological, biological, and sociological. Empathy, therefore, involves the worker's continuous efforts to fine-tune his/her understanding of the client in order to "get it right." Benjamin's ideas are based on an egalitarian model and provide the basis for the development of relationships that aim to minimize power differentials. Benjamin believes that when the client exerts a sense of agency and can see the clinician as a whole person, and when the practitioner can see the client as a whole person, the empathic encounter becomes truly alive. Although Lara and I came from different cultural worldviews, the mutual empathy that marked the helping process helped bridge our different backgrounds.

## Empathy and Empowerment: Yvette's Case

Since connections are important for self-definition and a sense of empowerment, creating the conditions that help others to use relational ties in constructive ways becomes a primary agenda for the practitioner. The following case vignette illustrates how as a social worker I used myself in a way that helped sensitize the client to the need to be empathic with others in her social environment. My relational orientation to practice fostered growth-promoting relationships on various levels—in the family, with the social worker in the mental health system, and with the case worker in the child welfare system.

When I was a psychiatric social worker in a court-affiliated mental health clinic, I was assigned the case of Yvette, a 36-year-old African-American woman diagnosed with schizophrenia. Yvette had a history of auditory hallucinations, for which she had been prescribed psychotropic medication. Prior to commencing treatment, Yvette terminated a long-term relationship with the father of her twin daughters. During this period she stopped taking her medication, which resulted in behavior of screaming and crying uncontrollably while her children were home. A neighbor called the police who took her to a hospital where she was admitted to the psychiatric unit. Her children were placed with the local child welfare agency. Pursuant to her discharge treatment plan, she saw me weekly at a local mental health center in addition to seeing a psychiatrist for medication.

When Yvette began counseling, her twins had been in foster care for two months. The focus of her treatment was twofold: 1) compliance with her medication regimen, and 2) working with the child welfare agency to achieve the return of her daughters. Initially, Yvette reported that her caseworker was cold, unfeeling, and "not on my side." She blamed the agency and "the system" for taking her children away from her. After two months of regular medication, Yvette's auditory hallucinations had considerably abated, she was working regularly, felt "ready to take care of my kids," and wanted them back. She was furious that the caseworker "wasn't helping me, wasn't doing her job, and didn't care about me or my kids." She wanted to call the worker's supervisor, contact the media, and "expose the system."

I encouraged Yvette to express her feelings, and empathized with her about her feelings of loss, rejection, and abandonment resulting from her romantic break-up and the loss of her children, whom she dearly loved. Prior to their removal, the children were relatively well cared for and doing well, despite their mother's difficulties.

After about one month, I said to Yvette, "I think that in order for you to get your children back you must understand the role, responsibilities, and feelings of your caseworker." At first, Yvette appeared not to understand, and seemed a little confused. "Why do I have to understand that bitch?" she asked. I responded, "Regardless of how you feel about her personally, you are intelligent enough to understand that the child welfare caseworker is the key to getting your kids back. Her recommendation carries a lot of weight, and unless she feels you are ready, it won't happen for a long time." I added, "I know you are upset, but I really want to try to help you get your daughters back. I would like you to just think about what I've said, and we'll continue to discuss this." In the interim, Yvette continued to visit her twins regularly.

During my next session with Yvette, I explained the role and responsibilities of the agency caseworker and emphasized the fact that if the agency returned the children to Yvette and they were harmed, the agency and the worker could be held responsible. I asked, "Do you think the worker wants her name in the newspaper if something happens to the kids she is supervising?" Yvette was quiet for a while and then said, "No, I guess not." I continued, "Do you realize that the caseworker could lose her job, and that she probably needs her job as much as you need yours?" Yvette was silent as she thought this over. In the next few sessions, I continued to explore Yvette's interactions with her child welfare worker. We even did some role plays together. Yvette reported that the caseworker had become increasingly friendly and more sympathetic to her, that she was taking her medication regularly, and that the auditory hallucinations had all but ceased. In December of 2006 the children were returned to Yvette under supervision.

The ability of the client to be empathic toward the worker shows his or her capacity and willingness to appreciate another person. Being empathic does not mean that the client necessarily identifies with the worker's personal concerns. Rather, recognizing that worker and client can be moved by similar feelings creates a shared experience, which then helps them construct a sense of commonality (Jordan, 1983).

This capacity to recognize the other not merely as an *object*, but rather as a *subject* is an important part of early development and life-long growth. Intersubjectivity and mutuality begin with the mother–child relationship. While it may be appropriate for the dependent infant to see the mother solely as a gratifying object, the relationship must eventually become more mutual if the child is to develop into a healthy adult. Winnicott (1965) terms this *the use of the object*, when the infant perceives the mother figure as not just a projection, but as an external reality, with her own wants and needs. As the child matures, the parent not only influences the child, the child also influences the parent. A parallel process takes place in the social work relationship.

## The Stone Center Approach to Empathy

Building upon the work of self-object/relational theorists such as Kohut and Winnicott, feminist theorists and practitioners from the Stone Center in Wellesley, Massachusetts, place the concept of empathy squarely at the center of human development (Jordan, 1989; Surrey, Kaplan, & Jordan, 1990). These scholars consider the worker's use of empathy essential in relationship building. As we previously saw with Lara, empathy provides a secure and safe context that maximizes the client's ability to feel free to be his/her authentic self. For these reasons, the power and value of empathy are highlighted in constructing a feminist relational paradigm for practice.

Stone Center scholars view empathy as a primary force that drives growth and development. Typically, it begins with mothers developing the capacity for empathy in their daughters through the process of same-sex role identification. Surrey et al. (1990) stress that, in most cultures, women live out their lives centered on the preparation for, and exercise of, a care-taking role. Early and continuous sex-role identification with a female figure, reinforced by gender-specific socialization processes, foster the capacity of females to be attuned to others (Chodorow, 1978). While both males and females are able to recognize and label the affective experience of another person (i.e. display cognitive awareness), Chodorow believes that females have been socialized to demonstrate a greater degree of responsiveness to others while most men have not been socialized to connect in quite the same way. Eisenberg et al. (1987) have conducted studies showing that gender differences develop because males and females are socialized differently. Similarly, Gilligan (1982) contends that girls and boys experience different paths of socialization, with girls being taught an ethic of caring rather than an ethic of justice. The difference becomes even more obvious in adolescence, when males are taught to "act out" (i.e. hide) their feelings when vulnerable (Hoffman, 1997).

## Boundary Management: Balancing Self-Autonomy with Affective Connection

Stone Center theorists equate empathy with sophisticated developmental and cognitive processes. Jordan (1983) views empathy as:

> an ability that requires a complex integration of cognitive and emotional capacities that provide a foundation for human connection . . . The affective component comprises feelings of emotional connectedness, a capacity to fully take in and contain the feelings of the other person. The cognitive component rests on one's integral sense of self and the capacity to act on the basis of that sense of self.
>
> (p. 13)

Jordan (1984) adds another dimension, stressing that empathy requires a complex integration of balancing cognitive and emotional capacities, providing the basic foundation for human connection. She suggests that empathy can be emotional *and* rational, affective *and* intellectual, and that the two can mutually co-exist. The challenge for the clinician is to empathize on an emotional level while exercising cognitive capacities needed to distinguish those feelings induced by the client as opposed to those feelings engendered by personal experience.

Belenky and her colleagues (1986) see the capacity for empathy, which they call "connected knowing," as a way to access another's way of thinking and feeling. They believe that since ideas come from experience, the only way to truly understand the other person's ideas is to attempt to understand the experience that led to their formation. This requires putting oneself in the place of the other and seeing the world from the other's perspective.

Connected knowing implies that empathy emerges through care, and caring represents a quest for understanding. People can only approximate another person's point of view, which necessitates that social workers ask questions in order to learn about their clients' culture, background, and the world in which they live (Belenky et al., 1986). Feedback from clients is the only way in which practitioners can be fully in tune with the client and adjust their perceptions accordingly. It is important to take risks, be genuine, be respectful, and be able to acknowledge when you are not being effectively empathic. You will know this if you reach for client feedback and if you are keenly tuned in to verbal and non-verbal cues. The deeper and more trusting the client–worker relationship, the more the client reveals, and the easier it is for the practitioner to see the world through the client's eyes.

Empathy requires a high level of cognitive structuring on the part of the social worker, who must simultaneously balance his/her own perception of reality with the meaning the client makes of a given situation. This requires an ability to oscillate from observer to participant, allowing the worker to "be" with the client without losing a sense of his/her own affective experiences. Oscillation between focusing on the self and focusing on the other takes skill, keen self-awareness, concentration, and boundary flexibility. It is this free flow of energy that is required for a true empathic exchange to occur.

Elements of emotional attunement and connected knowing coexist in every empathic encounter. Balancing affect and cognition is not always easy. For example, if the social worker and the client share the same experience or have a similar life history, over-identification may become an issue and a blurring of the boundaries might take place. While there may be a momentary overlap between self and other, the relational social worker rapidly shifts attention from the self to the client continuing to differentiate self from the other simultaneously and on an ongoing basis. In order to accomplish this level of mutuality, the worker must be grounded enough so as not to encourage closeness in order to gratify his or her own needs, or become too distant out of the fear of merger (Jordan, 1984).

Being able to feel deeply with another person suggests that one is able to temporarily suspend ego boundaries without the fear of losing oneself in the process. Contrary to past psychoanalytic notions wherein workers were overly concerned about maintaining emotional distance out of fear of encountering their own counter-transference reactions, the "relational" worker experiences and willingly expresses a wide range of thoughts and feelings, facilitating a sense of emotional connection with the client. Feeling deeply with another does not necessarily imply a form of "regressive merging," nor does it suggest a "blurring of the self." Rather, empathy is a sophisticated cognitive and emotional activity in which one person is able to experience the thoughts and feelings of another person as if they were one's own, while simultaneously being aware of the difference (Jordan, 1984). These ideas imply that the worker is mature and capable of maintaining a relatively clear sense of self and flexible ego boundaries to allow for the high degree of emotional and cognitive integration essential for empathy to be effective.

The power and value of empathic communication have been consistently recognized in social work literature as a tool used to enhance the helping relationship. Developing the capacity for empathy is a developmental goal, a dynamic part of the helping process, and a principal lever for change. In the Stone Center paradigm, the emphasis is placed on *mutual* empathy, which involves mutual participation and mutual action.

Feminist relational practitioners who aim to be authentic are active and expressive in their use of themselves. It is this critical ability to elaborate on one's own feelings and thoughts in the presence of another that allows for real engagement. Communication takes place through body language, facial expressions, affect, intonation, and reflection of manifest and latent content. When the worker responds in a genuinely empathic way, it is a kind of self-disclosure in which reactions are shared in the presence of the client. Distinct from the traditional approach, mutual empathy involves a conceptual shift—from a uni-directional technique in which the worker shows genuine concern, to bi-directional movement in which worker and client feel each other's active involvement and are engaged in genuine sharing.

## Mutual Empathy: Leslie's Case

The following case illustrates my attempt to establish a mutually empathic relationship with Leslie, whom we met in Chapter Three, now a 17-year-old high school junior.

As she approached her senior year in high school, Leslie increasingly expressed confusion and fear about going on to college. Leslie had lacked a stable home base for many years, so I was not surprised that leaving home again would be difficult. Having to make the decision about whether she was ready for college and which college to attend framed an identity crisis for Leslie similar to what most teens go through: Who am I? What do I want? Where do I belong? Will I make friends?

With my help, Leslie and her father researched different colleges and Leslie applied to several in the Midwest and Northeast. One day she proudly announced that she was accepted into two of them—a private college, her first choice, as well as an excellent state university. I felt very excited for Leslie and had a big smile on my face when I said, "I am so thrilled for you, Leslie, that is great news! What an accomplishment for you!" It was important that she really feel my happiness, since this moment was one of the most positive, life-affirming experiences Leslie had had in her recent past. When I asked her which school she was considering, she stated that although she was really happy to get accepted into both, she did not think her dad could afford the private college. Sensitive to her father's financial situation, Leslie said, "It would place an enormous burden on him, so I decided to accept the state university's offer. It's also closer to home."

At our next meeting, Leslie was able to share that not only was she disappointed about not going to the college she wanted most, but she also felt sad about not applying to the school near where her mother lived—her original intention. Having talked with her mom on the phone a few months earlier, Leslie realized that she was still neither sober nor stable. Leslie told me, "I am not ready to deal with her. It's best for me not to see or even talk to her at this point." She cried when I affirmed how painful it must have been for Leslie to realize that her dreams of going back home to her mom, family, and friends were shattered. I also let her know how important it is, even for adults, to want to share good news with the important people in our lives and how sad I was that now she couldn't even tell her mother. By creating an environment marked by respect and validation, I was providing Leslie with a place where she could fully be herself.

I was impressed with Leslie's growing sense of maturity and her ability to understand some of the realities upon which she based her decision and told her so. "Wow, I am really impressed with how much thought you have put into this decision and how mature you're being right now. I also know you are disappointed in giving up your dream school, but the State University is excellent and a great choice. I am really proud of you," I said. Leslie clearly felt my excitement and my pride in her accomplishments. She beamed and said that for the first time, she experienced a sense that someone actually cared about what *she* wanted instead of using her as a pawn for their own needs (referring to her parents).

Empathy is a quality that can lead to more fulfilling relationships. An emotionally healthy infant "tunes into" the mother's states of mind, not just to her behaviors (Beebe et al., 2002). As one matures, the ability to empathize on a higher level is one indicator of a healthy, integrated ego. Modeling this for the client does not necessarily mean disclosing personal information; rather, the worker is moved by the client's experience and responds accordingly. The client, in response, feels the worker's response, and knows that he or she has made an impact. In Leslie's situation I did share that I too had to attend a state university instead of the private one of my choice for financial reasons. With adolescents, the moment of mutual empathy often comes when you are genuine and "real" with them.

It is important to underscore that in the empathic exchange, the worker must truly experience the client's affective state in order to make an impact. In relational/cultural terms, this ability to feel deeply "with" the other person is called *affective resonance*. Affective resonance is a form of physiological arousal in which the worker experiences a vicarious emotional response while cognitively aware that the source of the feeling originates from the other person (Jordan, 1997a). The idea is for the client to feel that he/she has moved you, to know that there was an impact on you, and vice versa. The worker sometimes taps into memories of a similar situation of his/her own in order to intensify the connection, shifting back and forth between the worker's and the client's cognitive and affective processes. If successful, the empathic process is validating and deepens the sense of engagement between client and worker.

In my work with Leslie, it was particularly easy for me to communicate to her that she mattered and to join in her sadness. Given my belief that a female adolescent needs a strong sense of connection to her mother or mother surrogate to experience a well-differentiated sense of self, I felt particularly nurturing toward Leslie since her mother was unavailable to her. Furthermore, my ability to relate to her affective and cognitive state was deepened by the fact that she possessed qualities to which I could genuinely relate—a natural "earthy style," sensible values, and an interest in books and music of my generation.

Mutual empathy should not be confused with over-identification or counter-transference. Clearly, each person in the client–worker relationship has a different role and status, which serves to protect boundary integrity while allowing worker and client to feel connected to one another. According to Surrey et al. (1990), "Mutual empathy is not so much a matter of reciprocity—I give to you and then you give to me—but rather a quality of relatedness, movement, a dynamic of relationship" (p. 1).

While there may be a momentary surrender of feelings following affective cues, the worker should always maintain an awareness of the source of the feeling. Because, according to relational theory, movement and change happen through a matrix of connection, disconnection, and reconnection, the worker needs to be in touch with a vast array of thoughts and feelings that are in direct response to what the client is experiencing. Misunderstandings and differences, as well as connections and similarities that arise in the mutual flow, have to be negotiated and accepted for what they are in order for both the client and worker to grow (Surrey et al., 1990).

## On the Cultural and Political Side

The feminist-oriented relational approach has expanded its theoretical framework to include a heightened awareness of the diverse cultural and socio-political contexts that shape growth and development and relational experiences—what the Stone Center scholars refer to as a "relational–cultural approach to practice." The willingness to be genuinely empathic to another's worldview can provide a basis for a more collaborative relationship, one in which both worker and client can learn from their differences and well as from their similarities. Thus, cross-cultural empathy can help to deepen one's understanding of the client as well as to enhance a sense of mutuality.

This approach is based on the belief that any empathic connection cannot be fully realized without great sensitivity to the socio-cultural context in which the client is embedded. Gender-related experiences intersect with socioeconomic status, race, age, ethnicity, sexual orientation, and other forms of difference that situate people in a socially stratified society which then become powerful determinants of the reality of their lives (Jordan, Walker, & Hartling, 2004). Thus, if empathic communication is to be successful, it is critical that the worker understand that the client's worldview is filtered through a specific cultural frame of reference, including power differentials that exist across racial, ethnic, and gender lines.

The client's perception of power, or lack of power, is a critical ingredient in the worker's ability to establish a cross-cultural complementary helping relationship (Dyche & Zayas, 2001; Pinderhughes, 1979). The feminist relational school goes one step further to suggest that the social worker openly acknowledge the impact of cultural forces and power differentials. Knowing that resources and opportunities are often rewarded or withheld based on cultural privilege, it becomes important to bring power differentials and cultural determinants to the surface in an attempt to connect empathically with clients (Surrey et al., 1990).

The case of Joan illustrates this. Joan, a 45-year-old, Afro-Caribbean woman with whom I worked for two years, offers a good example of someone whose sense of empowerment increased in the context of our relationship, one marked by cultural sensitivity, mutual empathy, and respect. Joan had been a successful high-level bank executive for the past 12 years. However, she had recently been subjected to daily criticism from the newly hired bank president, a Caucasian male, who was connected to the "old boys' network" in the banking community. His insidious and constant belittling led her to believe that she was incompetent and that she had no other recourse but to leave her job. This kind of emotional abuse eroded Joan's self-esteem to the point that she initiated treatment, stating that her "world was falling apart."

Joan had dealt with discrimination previously in her career but did not expect it at this point, since she had been so successful and well-respected. We spent weeks exploring her feelings of shame and disappointment. I was deeply moved by and open to Joan's pain. As a female and as a professional, this resonated with experiences I have had in my own life and, in a general way, I let her know this. Joan saw that she had made an impact on me. I related that I felt sad that she was not able to change the image she had of herself based on the perceptions of a member of this society's dominant group (Collins, 1986). It was perhaps more disheartening for her to acknowledge extant racism and sexism than to blame herself for what she considered a "falling off" of her performance. And so she was left feeling helpless in the face of an oppressive force that she could not control.

When Joan discussed her work, she presented as articulate, bright, and clearly very competent. I was genuinely impressed with Joan's knowledge and skills and communicated my confidence in her by telling her this. I also reminded her that her sense of powerlessness and disconnection was exacerbated by the fact that she was culturally and socially isolated, since she was the only minority female bank executive at her workplace. Joan began to develop a heightened awareness of the social and political forces at play. A process of self-reflection unfolded, and she was able to explore alternative career opportunities. Eventually, Joan found another job in a work environment more compatible with her strengths and needs.

This kind of empathic connection established between worker and client can provide a blueprint that fosters the client's ability to form supportive, sustaining relationships beyond the helping one. Empathy can be viewed as the fuel or energy that drives the relational approach, and the client–worker relationship can be seen as the vehicle through which one experiences a basic sense of connection. An enhanced feeling of power can grow out of the healthy interaction with empathically attuned others contributing to the capacity to act in the environment with a greater sense of self-efficacy and purposefulness. Jean Baker Miller (1991b) calls this sense of being able to effect change in a larger relational context *agency-in-community*.

## Social Work Best Practices for Developing Empathic Relationships

As a social worker, you can strengthen empathic connections with clients through practicing a number of proven techniques. You can:

- *Intentionally seek intense emotional attunement*: attempt to feel the person's emotions as if they were your own. Start where the client is, allowing yourself to be vulnerable and open. Be attuned to the client, feeling with and validating their affective states, thoughts, and perceptions.
- *Create a relational image*: identify a situation in your own life, similar to the clients when similar feelings arose.
- *Share with clients only what is necessary*: selectively inform clients of your reactions, thoughts, feelings. Allow yourself to be known in ways that give the client helpful feedback and can allow them to feel that s/he has made an impact on you.
- *Open yourself to being affected by the other*: be authentic. Your responses should be congruent with the client's thoughts and feelings. Be aware that as two people connect, the distinction between them may blur.
- *Model authentic empathic attunement*: rather than being a passive repository, you may provide a reparative opportunity for earlier disconnections in which parts of the self were invalidated.

In summary, empathy is not just a technique, but is related to one's capacity for emotional connection. It allows for the existence of individual differences without the obliteration of individuality. Genuine empathy takes place in relational, cultural, economic, historical, and social contexts, and, hopefully, leads to an increase in the client's sense of well-being and sense of connectedness to others. The more connected clients feel to their social worker, the more they will open up and share information that the practitioner can use to develop an assessment and plan of intervention.

# 5 Assessment and Intervention
## A Relational Point of View

Since social work concerns itself with the person-in-environment as a way of understanding individuals and their problems, a relational assessment must include factoring in the context of family, friends, groups, community, the material and socioeconomic conditions that shape experience, the dimensions of identity, and society's response to those—race, ethnicity, gender, sexual orientation, religion, disability (Smith, Goodman, & Glenn, 2006). This chapter provides a framework for understanding how to conduct a relational assessment, what to include in a relational assessment, and possible points of intervention that flow from a relational viewpoint which integrates feminist scholarship and relational theory to best understand the person-in-environment.

Although a relational approach to assessment and the interventions that flow from it are not novel, the relational feminist orientation focuses more on *relationship* than other models in which relational variables may be secondary. Based on the theoretical framework developed by Stone Center practitioners/scholars at Wellesley College, this chapter examines relational processes, the structural components of relationships, and the implications of chronic disconnection within the context of family, group, and community.

## Assessment

There are many different types of assessments in social work practice: bio-psycho-social assessments, concrete-needs assessments, mental status exams, family assessments, and community and organizational assessments. In fact, assessment, which is the heart of social work practice and the foundation upon which our thinking and doing is based, is:

> The process of systematically collecting data about a client's functioning and monitoring progress on an ongoing basis. [It is a] process of problem selection and specification that is guided in social work by a person-in-environment orientation.
>
> (Levine, 2002, p. 830)

Good assessments and the decisions that follow involve the abilities to 1) amass and organize a variety of facts; 2) analyze the information together *with* the client; 3) understand the issues; and 4) determine the goals of the therapeutic process (Meyer, 1993).

According to Germain et al. (1996), assessment tasks common to most practice approaches include:

1    collecting data on life stressors and their degree of severity; the perception of the stressor; internal and external resources available for coping; cultural, biological, psychological, cognitive, familial, and environmental factors; and strengths and limitations;
2    organizing data in a way that reveals significant patterns and clarifies meaning;
3    analyzing and synthesizing data in order to draw inferences about strengths and limitations, environmental resources and deficits, and level of client–environment fit.

Feminist scholars Miller and Stiver (1997) at the Wellesley College Center for Research on Women have identified five growth-fostering relational characteristics that are helpful both in making assessments and evaluating outcomes: 1) mutuality, 2) a sense of empowerment, 3) a sense of self-worth and self-esteem, 4) a desire for more connection, and 5) the capacity to deal with inter-personal conflict. In addition, an evaluation of the client's capacities for engagement, authenticity, commitment, attunement, acceptance of diversity and difference, and mutual empathy can enhance the assessment and intervention process (Genero et al., 1992).

A relational assessment is a mutual, ongoing process that encourages clients' active participation in the collection of data and in thinking through the underlying forces and relational patterns that shape their experience. Clients are involved in the decision-making process to the fullest extent possible. This dynamic collaboration is used to enhance clients' awareness of self and others, and to evaluate their social supports, relationships, and available resources. The social worker who thinks relationally listens for clients' strengths, resources, and capacities, trying to find ways to capitalize on them. Sometimes this means helping clients to improve the quality of their relationships, to encourage new connections, or to help them extricate themselves from destructive relationships.

An effective relational assessment emphasizes relational connections— linkages as well as disconnections—not only for information and evaluation purposes, but also as a primary target for intervention. It pays close attention to the quality and quantity of relational structures and processes that exist in the client's life space. It is important to note that in the assessment process attention is paid to all relationships, past and present, across the client's life span. Individuals who are not physically present in the client's life are sometimes more significant than those who *are* physically present.

Thus, the visible (or sometimes invisible) thread of relational ties and connections or lack of connection to individuals, community, and social supports are important factors in assessment and intervention approaches. For example, a child in foster care who refuses to see his or her mother may indicate that exploration of this disconnection may be the initial point at which the social worker intervenes.

## The Paradox of Connection in a Relational–Cultural Context

The feminist–relational assessment in social work practice is embedded in a cultural context. Issues such as gender, power, domination, and subordination impact on client self-determination, access to institutional resources, and available opportunities for healthy connections. In the relational school of thought, the action of having power *over* is replaced by the idea of power *with*. The *power with*, or mutual power model, makes the development of empowering relationships central. Power *with* others connotes that each person is empowered through the relationship. The relationship then works to sustain mutual empathy and interest, which does not involve winning or losing but rather a commitment to deepen the connection (Surrey, 1987). I believe that a sense of empowerment comes from both inside and outside the individual. Individuals with a positive self-image and adequate self-esteem are more likely to have the energy and motivation to take action in their environment. Concurrently, the environment must provide the opportunities, concrete resources, and social supports that will allow clients to actualize their potentials and sense of empowerment. The relational worker focuses on the space in between—that context in which the interaction takes place.

A number of relational characteristics foster growth: 1) mutuality, 2) feeling empowered to take action, 3) gaining a greater sense of self-worth and validation, 4) an increased desire for more connection, and 5) the capacity to deal with conflict (Jordan, 1997b; Miller, & Stiver, 1997). A healthy sense of connection to others, in which the client feels truly listened to, understood, and respected, is an important source of empowerment. As suggested by Nancy Chodorow (1978), a sense of connection to others is *the* central organizing feature in women's development.

Culturally, it is generally more acceptable for females to seek out relationships and to stay connected longer and more intensively than males. The importance of social supports and relationships in women's health and adjustment has been well documented. Although there is a range of capacities for relationship among men as well as women, the research has supported what I have found in my own practice—that most males have more tenuous relational ties than most females, especially when it comes to close friendships (Kimmel, 2004). The challenge for the social worker is to help boys and men recognize the value of intimacy, and to encourage them to discover relational strategies for reaching out to others in authentic and growth-producing ways.

A brief case vignette demonstrates how I used the relational perspective as a way to develop an assessment of Tom, a 42-year-old Caucasian male who was caught in what Miller and Stiver (1997) have termed the "paradox of connection." This central paradox refers to a longing for affirming relationships, while the fear of connection keeps one from revealing his or her most vulnerable parts, thereby preventing true connection. Past trauma, loss, abandonment, and boundary violations may contribute to individuals' strategies to disconnect or hide parts of themselves from others in the home, family, school, community, etc. However, the clinical worker must remain empathic with both sides of the paradox, that is, the yearnings for connection as well as the methods used to stay out of connection.

I saw Tom and his wife Betty for marriage counseling for several months. Tom struggled to make a living as a construction worker. He was a skilled, experienced worker who spent long, hard hours at work. Yet he had not received a pay raise in the last two years, nor did he have the confidence to ask for one. His wife was dissatisfied because he did not make enough money for them to live comfortably. This hurt his pride, especially since other men he knew in their suburban community were better able to provide for their families. He felt a sense of humiliation at not being able to support his family in the life style his wife was accustomed to before their marriage.

Betty accused Tom of being an alcoholic, a charge that he denied. She was convinced that his drinking would destroy Tom, their marriage, and their family, which consisted of two small children, 7-year-old Johnny and 9-year-old Mary. Tom was often explosive at home. He had a particularly difficult relationship with Johnny with whom he was punitive and critical. Johnny was scared of his father's outbursts and Betty tried to protect him from her husband as best as she could. Betty's constant criticism and Tom's poor parenting skills only added to his sense of isolation and failure.

In addition, there seemed to be a great deal of disconnection between Tom and his family of origin. He saw his own parents occasionally but did not feel close to them, and he had virtually no relationship with his sister who lived in the Southwest. Weekends were usually spent with his mother-in-law with whom he had a poor relationship. When his wife brought up the fact that Tom was adopted in one of our sessions, he said, "It didn't really matter, and I don't want to talk about it." At this juncture in our work together, Betty decided to stop attending, and I continued to see Tom alone.

I believe Tom continued to see me in part because we had a good working relationship, in addition to the fact that he had no one else with whom he could talk. I commented that it did not seem as if he was connected with anyone in his life who made him feel good about himself. When I asked Tom if he had any friends with whom he enjoyed spending time, he simply said "no." However, he did mention that he used to "shoot hoops" with a buddy from high school but had not seen him in about five years. They just lost touch and had gone their separate ways. When I brought up the idea of reconnecting with his friend he was reluctant to do so. Alienated from his family and friends, the only real connection he had was to alcohol. In his struggle to shut out pain and disappointment he retreated into his own world, numbing his feelings and oblivious to the feelings of others.

Looking at this case from a relational point of view, I realized that Tom lacked relational awareness and had few satisfying relationships except for the therapeutic one we had established together. According to Judith Jordan (2004), "relational awareness is not about analyzing relationships. It involves an attitude of openness to learning about relational patterns" (p. 54). For Tom, being open and accessible to others was a sign of weakness. Uncertain of his own identity, ashamed of his economic plight in life, feeling excluded by his family, he was like an egg with a fragile shell, desperate to protect himself from shattering. Consequently, Tom allowed himself few meaningful interpersonal connections so as not to risk piercing his emotional barrier.

Tom, like other individuals who do not feel valued or powerful, would sometimes self-isolate; at other times, he displaced his anger and shame onto his family. Paradoxically speaking, Tom desired relational connections as was demonstrated by his commitment to his family. However, under stress, his strategy was to become aggressive or to disconnect. He would not permit himself to be vulnerable or to express his needs. Nor would he allow himself to explore his feelings and thoughts about his adoption. His disconnection from important parts of his history led me to wonder how much intimacy he could really tolerate.

As with Tom, I believe that behind most personal problems lay chronic disconnections, violations, or distorted images of self and other. Sometimes the precipitating factors that create tension and maladaptive behaviors are rooted in environmental stress; most of the time they result from an interlocking of inner and outer forces. An important role for the social worker is to assist clients with establishing healthier and more trusting relationships that may result in more effective psycho-social functioning.

Jean Baker Miller and Irene Stiver (1997) identify five beneficial components—what they call "five good things"—that result from relationships characterized by empathy, honesty, and respect:

1   an increased sense of zest or well-being that comes with feeling connected to others;
2   the motivation to put feelings and thoughts into words and action;
3   an increased knowledge about oneself and others;
4   an increased sense of self-worth; and
5   a desire for more connection.

The social worker who is knowledgeable about these "five good things" can help the client develop optimal relationships, which can lead to a greater sense of self, the motivation to be a more active agent in the environment, and enhanced self-esteem—outcomes central to and consistent with the goals of social work practice and feminist ideology.

Frequently, there are obstacles in relationships that impede the achievement of the "five good things," those "things" being a complex mix of elements that can easily be converted into negative consequences if we are involved in relationships that incur shame, violation, or trauma, resulting in a negative sense of self. The problem develops at the interface—the common contact barrier where interaction occurs. This meeting place symbolizes each person's sense of being with the other, accompanied by the other's feelings and thoughts. What starts as a problem in the interaction often becomes internalized as a problem originating in the person and may be experienced as a personal failing. Women and girls in particular have been socialized to look to others for affirmation and value, placing them in a more vulnerable position to external criticism than boys and men (Surrey, 1987).

## Self-Esteem

An important question to ask oneself in making an assessment is: does this particular relationship give the client energy and power or does it deplete self-esteem and obstruct growth and development? Power and self-esteem are closely connected. People feel diminished when they are labeled in negative ways. However, when a person feels validated, accepted, respected, his or her sense of self flourishes, mobilizing inner resources for both problem solving and goal attainment. According to Jordan (1994), relational mutuality—mutual respect, mutual empathy, relatedness—can provide purpose and meaning in individuals' lives, while a lack of it can adversely affect self-esteem. Germain's (1991) definition of self-esteem fits well with the relational model: "positive feelings about oneself acquired through experiences of relatedness, competence, and self-direction across the life course" (p. 26).

Traditional views suggest that our sense of competence and overall self-image is based on how we stack up against others. In other words, how we evaluate ourselves has to do with how we meet certain social and cultural ideals and standards set by our families, peers, mentors, community, and the larger society. The opinion others have of us is often internalized and incorporated into our self-esteem without our conscious awareness—particularly so with women. Sometimes there is synchrony between individuals' beliefs and societal values and sometimes not, creating conflict and possible shame (Walker, 2004).

Competition is encouraged in bureaucracies like school systems and work places, where the hierarchical arrangement of power serves to get people to work harder. In this "separate self" model, an individual's sense of well-being can be derived from comparing one's self to others, and judging that self to be "better." These values of individual achievement and self-sufficiency are antithetical to the values of collaboration and connection rooted in the relational model.

The following case illustrates how a competitive mother–daughter relationship and a competitive school environment can undermine the ability to develop a realistic and positive sense of self, contributing to feelings of low self-esteem and disempowerment.

## Anna's Case: Background and Assessment

Anna, a 20-year-old Caucasian college student from the West Coast, was enrolled in a dance conservatory program in the East Coast. She came to see me after her first episode of major clinical depression. Anna had lost 25 pounds, was listless, and had stopped attending classes. Her psychiatrist prescribed anti-depressant medication and advised her to take a six-month leave of absence from school. The college required that Anna receive weekly counseling as a condition of re-instatement.

During the first session, Anna seemed extremely self-conscious. She stated that she continuously judged herself in comparison to her classmates—she was either "much better" or "much worse." She strove for perfection, and felt that anything that fell short of that standard was unacceptable to her.

Anna's mother, Mrs. J., was also a dancer and choreographer who had given dance lessons since Anna was young. Consequently, Anna had to compete for her mother's approval and attention with hundreds of other girls. She wanted to "stand out" and "be recognized" for her unique talents. Unfortunately, she never felt she succeeded. Anna's younger sister was also training to be a dancer. Her father, Mr. J., was a salesman and mostly concentrated on making a living for the family.

As she approached adolescence, Anna began to feel particularly vulnerable to rejection and ridicule. She stated that she felt different from others her age in her school and community because of her "artsy" way of dressing and her non-conformist behavior. Afraid that she would be judged as "weird" by the other girls, she spent much of her time alone. The specialized performing arts college Anna attended was highly competitive, thereby intensifying the pressure she felt to succeed in the "real world" of dance. This atmosphere exacerbated Anna's anxiety and depression, leading her to further isolate and distance herself from her peers. She was in constant competition to prove to herself and, I suspect, to her mother that she was worthwhile. Even though her mother was miles away, Anna had internalized her critical voice.

## Anna's Case: Analysis and Discussion

The very continuity of mother–daughter ties allows for growth and maturation. However, there must be room for conflict and questioning, leading not to separation, but to self-differentiation (Kaplan, Klein, & Gleason, 1985). The mother–daughter relationship can be the basis for a positive relational mode of development. However, the child must be secure with herself and the relationship if she is to take a step toward changing the relationship in more complex and developmentally appropriate ways without disrupting underlying qualities of care and commitment. It seemed that Anna had had some doubts about her career in dance that she could not openly acknowledge for fear of her mother's disappointment. It appeared that Mrs. J. had a difficult time accepting Anna unconditionally, and did not project the kind of confidence in her that Anna could incorporate into a positive image. Anna felt afraid that she would lose her mother's love and approval if her performance wasn't "perfect" or if she doubted her ability and desire to dance. Most of Anna's judgment of herself had been based upon her mother's real or imagined approval or disapproval of her performance, and therefore the physical separation from home intensified Anna's doubts about her abilities.

Faculty members can be a source of personal validation for students and they become an integral part of their human connection at school. Unfortunately, Anna felt that she did not get adequate feedback from the teacher whose work she admired and respected the most. How could I help Anna build a more mutually supportive relational context in which she felt enough safety and care to bring more of her own self into authentic connections with others? How could I help her to be less harsh and more accepting of herself?

## Anna's Case: Intervention Strategies

My overall plan was to help Anna feel more competent, increase her self-esteem and self-direction, and help her to connect to others in more mutually satisfying ways. I asked Anna about her own performance standards, hoping to place more of the locus of control with her. I empathized with the reality of the stress that she was feeling and validated the nature of the competitive world in which she was immersed, hoping this would increase her confidence and mitigate some of her self-criticism.

The turning point in the helping process came when Anna was chosen to be in the Spring Dance concert and asked me if I would attend. After hearing how important it was to her, I decided to go. Since her parents could not come, as they lived 3,000 miles away, I thought it was particularly significant for Anna to have someone there just for her. Afterwards, she asked me if I enjoyed the show. I shared my genuine pleasure in seeing her perform and told her how much I liked the production. Anna said that she was honestly surprised that I did not see the major mistake that she made at the beginning of her performance. She acknowledged that perhaps it was her own self-consciousness and unrealistic expectations that made her so unforgiving and hypercritical of herself; she expected either perfection or criticism—nothing in between.

However, I sensed some disconnection between us at this point in the process, and so I asked Anna how she felt when I said that I did not notice her mistake. She stated that she did not feel I was as observant or astute as someone who was trained in dance, and that therefore I would not have noticed her mistake. I shared with Anna that I felt she was devaluing my feedback in part because she was so harsh on herself. I put her message into words for her: "How could anyone who had good sense think my perform-ance was good?" I let Anna know that her dismissal of me made me feel devalued. She said she felt sad she hurt my feelings, and did not want to be mean to me. She was quite empathic at that moment and I was moved by this.

I felt that Anna was being dismissive of me but was even more cruel to herself for not being able to take in a "good object," because to do so might display disloyalty to her mother. After this mutually honest exchange, I believe that Anna trusted me enough to take in the positive feedback I offered. Now the challenge is for Anna to integrate a more realistic and positive self-concept as she moves into adulthood.

Anna made an interesting comment toward the end of our next to last session before she was to return home for the summer. She said that although she knew she was intellectually bright, she has always felt her social intelli-gence was below par. It has always been hard for her to feel empathy for others or to relate to people with interest and care. But through our relation-ship she began to connect more to her own feelings and to cultivate empathy for others. During one session after I had seen her performance Anna said, "You know, I might even want to be a dance therapist so I can help others. I can't believe I can actually feel with others. I was never able to do that before." Slowly, Anna had begun to develop a greater self-acceptance of herself and a less critical self-introject.

## The Importance of Relational Connections and Contexts

Jean Baker Miller (1986) suggests that self-worth is a natural by-product of girls' and women's effectiveness in establishing, participating in, and main-taining mutually gratifying relationships. A shift in relational connections can be critical in realigning supports, creating a spiral of positive feelings and an increased sense of strength in the agential self. In contrast to a sense of well-being, situations that contribute to low self-esteem are characterized by the sense of being unable to create movement or change.

The capacity to engage in a satisfying relationship with another person does not preclude the sense of accomplishment that arises after completing a task successfully. Robert White (1963) theorized that humans possess an inborn drive toward mastery and competence. However, in order to achieve positive feelings about oneself the environment must provide the necessary conditions, opportunities, resources and relationships. The following is a list of ways practitioners may enhance the well-being and psycho-social func-tioning of clients while building self-esteem:

1   Explore the client's access to relationships that are responsive to his or her unique characteristics and temperament.
2   Help clients identify, establish, and expand relationships characterized by empowerment, empathy, genuineness, and responsiveness.
3   Encourage clients to identify and seek relationships that contribute to their learning opportunities and intellectual development, e.g. with mentors and teachers.
4   Assist clients to locate opportunities to enhance their sense of competence.
5   Explore clients' opportunities to create connections through peer groups, community groups, and self-help groups.
6   Examine the ways in which clients can make meaningful contributions to others through social action, mentoring, and community service.
7   Share feedback at moments of connection and disconnection between client and worker, and between client and external world.

## Relational Inventories

The quality and properties of one's social ties, social networks, community linkages, and personal relationships can allow for more effective problem solving and the ability to deal with societal inequities, feelings of powerlessness, and low self-esteem. A number of research studies are available that can help the worker evaluate the importance of relationships and social supports in women's lives. The Relational Health Indices (RHI) (Laing et al., 1998) is one example of an exploratory study that is designed to assess growth, fostering peer, mentor, and community relationships based on the relational/cultural theory set forth by feminist scholars at the Wellesley College Stone Center. The Relational Health Indices (RHI) was administered to a group of 450 first-year and senior students at a women's liberal arts college. The research design includes a set of three scales that assesses mentoring relationships, peer relationships, and community relationships separately. In particular, the concepts of self-disclosure and openness, authenticity, empowerment/zest, and the ability to deal with difference or conflict, were found to be associated with growth-fostering relationships.

The quality of one's connection to community, peers, and mentors was predictive of depression and loneliness scores. Self-esteem was associated with all three relational types. This is important information because it suggests that the social worker needs to pay attention to those relationships that 1) are mutual and respectful, 2) can facilitate emotional resiliency and coping strategies, and 3) provide motivation for reaching out for additional social supports. Furthermore, the relational scales developed to measure these nuanced qualities represent directions for future research that can be administered to populations such as low-income women who find themselves in the shelter system, young men in the juvenile justice system, and teen mothers without partners.

I adapted the following questions from the Relational Scale Question-naire (RSQ) developed by Griffin and Bartholomew (1994). I often use these as a semi-structured open-ended questionnaire at various stages of the assessment process to help focus the interview on gathering informa-tion that may shed light on the nature and quantity of mutual satisfying relationships:

1  Are there people in your life on whom you feel you can depend?
2  Are there people in your life who you feel can depend on you?
3  How important is it for you to feel independent?
4  How comfortable are you depending on other people?
5  How easy is it for you to get emotionally close to another person?
6  How comfortable are you with being alone?
7  Do you think you get as much as you give in your close relationships?
8  Do you think your relationships are characterized by mutual interest and respect?
9  Do you think that others value you as much as you value them?
10  Do you feel you are able to express your feelings, thoughts, and opinions clearly?
11  Do you feel you are listened to?
12  Do you feel you listen to the other person's point of view?
13  Are others energized by their relationship with you?
14  Do you feel supported and encouraged in your close relationships?
15  Do you feel you are able to give support and encouragement to others?
16  Do you feel you can be genuine and real in your close relationships?
17  Do you feel others are honest and real with you?
18  Do you feel you are able to negotiate difference and conflict in your relationships?
19  Do you feel you are open to accepting and dealing with conflict and differences in your relationships?

In my work with Anna, her responses to these questions were enlightening for me, but for Anna as well. She was able to see more clearly that her lack of connectedness with others in the campus community left her without a sense of belonging, which contributed to her loneliness and depression. Her characteristic style of relating was to use distancing maneuvers related to her anxiety about how she would be judged by others.

Think of an individual with whom you work. Imagine you are that per-son. How do you think he or she would answer these questions? What additional information might you gather from his or her responses that would guide your intervention techniques? Cultural arrangements and power practices can divide people into groups of dominants and subordinates (Jordan et al., 2004). An analysis of cultural concepts may range from the use of power in a patriarchal society to issues of racial identity and growing up as a member of a minority group in which one's experiences are affected by gender, class, race, age, ethnicity, sexual orientation, and other markers that evoke oppression.

Assessing levels of felt marginalization and recognizing difference and diversity are intrinsic to a relational assessment. For example, groups and individuals that deviate from the dominant culture's ideals are devalued by the larger society. In turn, signs of withdrawal, lack of motivation to act on the environment, anger, and even despair may be manifested. This dynamic exerts a powerful influence on how people interact with others and may even create a vicious cycle of marginalization (Surrey, 1987). Clients from diverse cultural, economic, ethnic, racial, and other social groupings who have experienced oppression, marginalization, and prejudice may view the social worker (and the agency) with skepticism. This too should be factored into the assessment process.

The following case illustrates the lack of connection between a 15-year-old African-American adolescent and the primary social systems with which she interacted—family, school, and peers.

## The Case of Lisa: A Relational/Cultural Context

Lisa's mother, Mrs. M., called the counseling center requesting help for her daughter, whom she described as moody, explosive and unhappy. Furthermore, Mrs. M. was concerned about Lisa's grades, poor study habits, and lack of organizational skills. I initially met with Lisa and her mother together. Mrs. M. is an attractive 48-year-old woman who appears both self-assured and somewhat anxious at the same time. Lisa is a moderately overweight, pleasant teen who is quite engaging. She is a bright, articulate teen who displayed keen insight into herself and others.

Mrs. M. expressed resentment about Lisa's lack of consideration of others at home, stating that "she leaves the house a mess and never picks up after herself." Mrs. M. feels that her daughter makes excessive demands on her life; particularly in relation to her school work and social needs. Mrs. M. is a special-education teacher and is very invested in Lisa's school success. However, she states that Lisa does her homework "at the last minute" and then wants help from her mother late at night. Mrs. M. also stated that Lisa is intrusive when Mrs. M. has friends over, leaving her little time for her own life. She wants Lisa to get involved in extracurricular activities at school, and to socialize with friends her own age. In essence, Mrs. M. feels that Lisa is too dependent on her for her social and emotional needs.

Lisa feels that her mother does not listen to her, validate her feelings, or understand her needs and wants. Lisa admits that she has a hard time concentrating and thus procrastinates when it comes to doing her school work. She sees it as a problem and wants her mother to understand and empathize with her frustration rather than blame her for not doing well in school. Lisa is angry with both of her parents. Mr. M. is a detective in the police force and is often at work or out of the house with his friends. When he is at home he is emotionally unavailable and usually ignores Lisa. Lisa resents his lack of involvement in her life and verbalized that she would like to do more things with her father. Mrs. M. also feels the lack of her husband's presence, since much of the burden of rearing Lisa falls on her shoulders.

Lisa agreed to see me individually on a weekly basis. In fact, she seemed quite eager to talk to someone. From time to time I saw Lisa with her mother and on a few occasions I saw Lisa with her father. Lisa fears that her parents, after being together for 15 years, will get divorced. Although she is aware that they share little physical affection or emotional intimacy, she enjoys the comfortable middle-class lifestyle, material possessions, and the sense of family they have been able to maintain. She says, "I don't want to be like my other friends who live in the housing development near my house and come from single parent families."

According to Lisa, her interest in academics and middle-class life style distance her from some of her peers who see her as "un-cool" and "too white." Lisa is quite aware that she lives in a racist society where the majority culture has constructed stereotypes about black youth. Patricia Hill Collins refers to this idea as the concept of "controlling images" imposed by the dominant culture to define and marginalize subordinate groups (Jordan et al., 2004). These "images" often evoke race, gender, sexual orientation, or ethnicity. Lisa talks freely with me about the fact that she feels some of her teachers discriminate against the black kids and favor the white and Hispanic kids. She doesn't feel comfortable going to these teachers for extra help and, not surprisingly, she is doing most poorly in the classes in which she is receiving the most parental pressure—Math and English.

In middle school it was easier for Lisa to have relationships with youngsters from diverse backgrounds, but in high school it has become more difficult as the girls self-group based on social markers such as race, economics, ethnicity, and sexual orientation. Furthermore, as Lisa moved into her middle teens her attempt to establish a personal identity was more intertwined with her racial identity, and there are few middle-income African-American students in her school with whom she can identify. In order to cope with her fear of rejection and social discomfort, she cuts herself of from school activities and heads home alone after school to "unwind."

During our subsequent sessions Lisa reiterated many of the same problems she stated in our beginning sessions—her distant relationship with her father, her strained relationship with her mother, whom she experiences as withholding and critical, and difficulty with her school work. She feels that her parents put great pressure on her to achieve at school and she does not want to share with them that she is having a particularly difficult time in her Math and English classes.

A crisis erupted after I had been seeing Lisa for a couple of months. Mrs. M. phoned in a very agitated state to tell me that Lisa had forged her signature on two English tests that she had failed. When I met with Lisa she, too, was clearly upset. She said, "I want to understand why I do what I do."

She recognized that forging her mother's signature on her English tests was a way to avoid her parents' disapproval and was also perhaps a cry for help.

This incident seemed to open the way for Lisa to share thoughts and feelings she had kept to herself for many years. She related that she felt unwanted and that no one would care if she were dead or alive. She feels responsible for her parents' troubled relationship. Although her mother denies this and claims that Lisa was premature, Lisa told me that her parents only married because of her mother's pregnancy with her. This was and still is a family secret.

## Analysis and Discussion

Lisa lives in a lonely, confusing world in which she feels misunderstood. She experiences her parents as non-responsive to her needs and experiences, which negates the legitimacy of her feelings and beliefs. Lisa's parents, by their own account have an "empty" marriage, which contributes to a household that is devoid not only of joy, but also of hopeful connection. The difficulties Lisa's parents have with one another make her sad.

Every family has its share of secrets. However, secrecy denies unacceptable realities that contribute to patterns of systemic and chronic disconnections among family members (Miller & Stiver, 1997). Not only did the secret of her mother's pre-marital pregnancy cause Lisa to feel unwanted and responsible for the family problems, it also left her feeling isolated because she experiences her parents as emotionally inaccessible. Her strategy for dealing with these feelings within the home is to alternate between being "clingy," and being angry and explosive.

The sense of secrecy surrounding the family contributes to Lisa's sense of isolation and disempowerment. There seems to be a pact in the family, which creates a denial of reality for Lisa, and a denial of her own inner experience: "Let's act like we are a family even though we are all disconnected from one another and mom and dad really don't love each other." This need to hide their relationships causes Lisa's family to turn away from relationships with other community institutions such as the church, girl scouts, school activities, and committees. Lisa's strategy to deal with her unhappiness outside of the home is to further cut herself off from large parts of her social world, in particular, peers her own age, and to disconnect from school.

In this family, the lack of intimacy and mutuality between Mr. and Mrs. M. affects all of the family members, especially Lisa. Not having the opportunity to construct an open, mutual relationship with her parents exaggerates the normative power inequities that typically exist between adolescents and their parents, leaving Lisa feeling helpless. For example, while Lisa has a great need to be understood, her mother and father expend so much energy on trying to keep their relationship together for the sake of appearances, that it is difficult for them to be responsive to Lisa. Especially significant is the fact that Mrs. M. is a wonderful role model in many ways, but Lisa doesn't believe she can win her approval. In order to feel more powerful, Lisa is often angry and rude with her parents, teachers, and peers, causing them to withdraw from her. She is acutely aware of this interactional pattern and told me that although she doesn't want to change the essence of who she is, she would like to "soften" her "edges."

A supportive parent–child relationship is characterized by expressions of warmth and the absence of harsh criticism, and expressions of affection and good communication (Rutter, 1990). Interestingly, research findings show that major factors contributing to resilience in children and youth growing up in families characterized by marital discord have to do with the importance of relationships outside the family (Werner, 1989). Lisa has a loving and close relationship with her paternal grandparents who give freely of their time and money. This relationship compensates for the less than optimal one with her parents and supplies her with the protective factors predictive of her resilience. This mutually nurturing and caring relationship provides Lisa with a different relational image of herself and allows her to maximize her social potentials, her intelligence, her caring, and her warmth.

## Relational Intervention Strategies

I asked Lisa to write her thoughts, feelings, and experiences in a journal as a means of getting to know herself better and to help me to know her better. She allowed me to read her journal every week, and it provided a wonderful vehicle for us to connect in a meaningful and non-threatening way. One day I asked her to tell me about her friends, who seemed noticeably absent in her journal. This question segued into a discussion about the kinds of "friends" she has. Although she hangs around with some kids in school, Lisa admits that they are more like acquaintances than a cohesive group of good friends in whom she can confide or trust. We spent some time talking about what creates a sense of closeness and trust with others, and what creates a sense of distance and mistrust in friendships. Some of the questions I posed to her were: How do you respond to your friends' needs? How do you show your friends you care and understand? How do your friends respond to your needs? How do they show you they care? Do you feel they understand you? Is your interest in each other reciprocal? Lisa and I discussed the importance of her listening to others and having friends who are able to listen to her, willing to be there for her when she needs them, and vice versa.

Lisa was open to engaging with me in a therapeutic relationship and was willing to confront the issues in her life. I helped her to develop some ways to express her feelings and thoughts to her parents when she felt they were not listening to her or understanding her. Reclaiming her voice in a more appropriate manner helped reduce some of her depression and frustration. I also referred Mr. and Mrs. M. to another social worker in my agency for couples' counseling. After a few sessions, they decided not to continue due to the fact that Mr. M. was unmotivated to make changes in the relationship. However, Lisa eventually came to understand that she did not "cause" whatever problems exist between her parents.

Lisa stated that she wanted to do more things with her father. Mr. M. agreed to come in for a session with Lisa and me, during which Lisa was able to share her feelings directly with him. During the session Mr. M. was able to listen to Lisa and to admit that he often brings home his frustration and anger from his very stressful job. I helped Lisa to integrate this information so that she doesn't take her father's moods personally. Mr. M. seemed to want to improve his relationship with Lisa and they made a date to go bowling. She was thrilled with this arrangement.

Next I met with Lisa and her mother. Both of them were willing to work on their relationship. They know that they need to listen to each other more carefully rather than to get defensive and "hotheaded" with each other. I talked with Mrs. M. about the importance of being more empathic with Lisa—listening to Lisa more carefully and to trying to understand what she is feeling. I appealed to the mother's strengths as a teacher who is sensitive to her students' needs, hoping to harness those same strengths, which will allow her to be more empathic and accepting of Lisa. Lisa, on the other hand, must develop greater empathy for her mom in order to strengthen their bond and make it a truly mutual one. This will make it easier for Lisa to establish a secure base with mom from which to differentiate herself and establish her own identity.

Through our relationship, Lisa was able to appreciate the value of other relationships in her life. She rekindled a friendship with her cousin who lives a short distance away. Lisa is motivated to do well in school and to go to college in North Carolina where her maternal grandparents live. I let her know how intelligent and insightful I think she is, how much I enjoy working with her, and how I love her beautiful smile. My feedback gave her tremendous encouragement and inspired her to try harder. For example, with my support Lisa decided to seek Math and English help in summer school. With the help of tutors her mother procured for her, she was very pleased with the fact that she earned an A and a B for her summer courses.

## Social Work Best Practices for Assessment, Planning, and Intervention

As a social worker you can enhance to assessment process through practicing the following techniques. You can:

- Systematically explore and reach for clients' feelings about those significant relationships in which there has been a disconnection. Keep in mind that those relationships which are absent from a person's life my be more clinically relevant than those which are present.
- Be proactive in enabling clients to become mutual partners in the

assessment process. A dynamic collaboration process works best in achieving system goals.

- Assess levels of felt marginalization and recognize that difference and diversity are intrinsic to a relational assessment. Sensitivity to cultural diversity must be factored into a relational assessment; the ability to be self-reflective affects the worker's ability to gather data, analyze data, assess the person-in-situation configuration, and derive goals and a plan of action.
- Establish linkages to social networks in the community to reduce isolation and maximize the opportunities for healthy, growth-producing connections. The worker's action must be directed toward assessing the nature and quality of social supports, and where necessary, mobilize institutional resources, community programs and organizations, that will support and enhance the client's coping and adaptive capacities.
- Use your assessment to evaluate the degree to which the client would benefit from the expression and fulfillment of dependency needs in various life's relationships and under various circumstances, including the professional one. Assess the degree to which the client would benefit from striving toward more self-directed, autonomous functioning.

In summary, assessing the clients relationships in their total life space can help impact upon their self-esteem, sense of worth, and their ability to experience themselves as effective and impowered individuals within their life space.

# 6 Ethics and Values
## A Relational Perspective

Every practice paradigm in social work is supported by a constellation of values and a code of ethics that are reflected in the mission, theoretical and empirical base, practice skills and techniques, and general philosophy and outlook of that paradigm. These ethics and values are not merely abstract concepts—they hold everyday importance for all social workers. A brief overview of the values and ethics that guide the feminist-relational approach to practice will incorporate most of the themes presented in this book.

Feminist ethics and values have utility for social work and are reflected in the National Association of Social Workers' *Code of Ethics*, which provides the standards of behavior for social work practice. For example, values emerging from feminist-relational theory challenge the dominant society's accepted or implicit ideas about race, gender, sexual orientation, and class, as well as focus change efforts on ensuring rights and equality for every oppressed and culturally/ethnically diverse group (Sands & Nuccio, 1992).

Professional values and ethics, which share important principles with philosophical systems of feminism, have an impact on almost everything we do; what we ask, how we intervene, and how we interpret what we find. Values and ethics are the underpinnings of the social work profession and play an important role in how social workers respond to situations, make decisions, and enact their roles on a day-to-day basis (Phillips & Straussner, 2002). The NASW *Code of Ethics* is "based on the fundamental values of the social work profession that include the worth, dignity, and uniqueness of all persons as well as their rights and opportunities" (p. 1). Three core values identified in the Code and also given particular attention in the feminist relational model are:

1    the inherent worth and dignity of the human being;
2    mutual respect, acceptance, and caring; and
3    self-determination.

## The Inherent Worth and Dignity of the Human Being

Feminist values of interdependence and interconnectedness, relational commitment, and a morality that encompasses mutual compassion and care correspond to the social work value that has perhaps the most consensus in the field: "the vision of the unique individual with inherent dignity, sharing common needs with others" (Collins, 1986, p. 216). Since its inception, social work has had to justify its value base to other male-dominated professions that regard caring as "unscientific" and merely an extension of the female role (Freedberg, 1993).

There are few fixed rules in the practice of social work. Ethical systems must take into account culture, context, personality, the nature of the client–worker relationship, and the nature of the client's connections. Particular responses reflecting ethical thinking are individualized for social work's increasingly diverse clientele.

Perhaps most central to the feminist relational perspective is the notion, discussed in Chapter Three, of *mutuality*, a unifying concept that underlies both the practice and the ethics of social work. Genero and her colleagues (1992) refer to mutuality as "the bi-directional movement of feelings, thoughts, and activity between persons in relationships" (p. 36). This suggests an openness to the constant changing patterns of worker and client responding to and affecting each other's state, with a special awareness of the other's subjective experience (Jordan, 1986). Simply stated, when one is the recipient of concern, attention, and care, one is in a better position to give these back, thereby enhancing the quality of all of one's relationships.

Empathy combined with mutuality allows the worker to get a sense of how the client thinks and feels, so that together worker and client can co-create a shared relational experience. Surrey (1997) states that "Mutuality describes a creative process, in which openness to change allows something new to happen, building on the different contributions of each person" (p. 42). Encouraging a sense of mutuality maximizes feelings of competence, which leads to an increased sense of worth and dignity. In sum, mutuality entails mutual appreciation, communication, sharing, and the commitment of each being there for the other. With the ongoing experience of relationships characterized by mutuality and relational bonding, real care and concern emerge.

We do not live in a world that always respects mutuality. Whenever one group of people has power over another, disconnections and violations can result. The mutuality model, in contrast to the power-over model, aims to enhance the individual's self-respect and supports the worth and dignity of each human being by bringing action and awareness to opposing oppression. All oppression is relational, acting *against* mutuality and thus creating major rifts between groups.

The motivation to connect *with* others, rather than to merely be gratified *by* others, represents a basic shift from traditional approaches (Miller &

Stiver, 1997). Mutuality offers each person an opportunity to contribute actively at different levels, minimizing power differentials and enhancing self-respect and self-esteem. How we, as social workers, share our mistakes and how we handle our own uncertainties can increase trust and minimize unnecessary power imbalances that detract from the dignity of the client.

When the practitioner's belief in authenticity, mutuality, and empathy are seen as an essential component of effective social work, the client is protected to some degree from exploitation, although complete psychological safety can never be assured. In relationships in life outside the helping relationship of client–worker, when caring individuals assist each other to disengage from unhealthy connections that erode self-esteem, these healthy forms of connection (Jean Baker Miller's "five good things") lead to positive outcomes including increased zest; increased desire and ability to act; increased knowledge of self and others; increased sense of self-worth; and a desire for more connection. Thus, a relational framework linked to the importance of mutuality plays itself out not only in the therapeutic client–worker relationship, but between clients and their friends, work colleagues, significant others, parents, and children.

## Mutual Respect, Acceptance, and Caring

Mutuality involves being engaged in a growing connection with another person. As the relationship unfolds, honoring the uniqueness of each other becomes integral to the growth of mutual respect. Reflection can be used to identify, explore, and affirm a client's strengths, abilities, and uniqueness. The social work practitioner acts as an empathic investigator, revealing the client's self to the client, and then engaging him or her in a relationship in which each enjoys being part of the experience, feeling *with* the other, being moved, being understood, and being accepted by the other.

Social work is also about care. In fact, caring about others is considered the very foundation of social work (Rhodes, 1985). Psychologist and philosopher Willard Gaylin (1978) defines caring as:

> the protective, parental, tender aspects of loving is a part of relationship among peers, child to parent, friend to friend, lover to lover, person to animal. The parent-child aspect of caring is the only essential paradigm whose presence is necessary for the diffusion of this human quality into the other relational aspects of life.
>
> (p. 33)

It is difficult to define *care* in absolute terms, but it would seem to be related to an act of well doing, a moral obligation, or the responsibility to be there for another. Caring can be perceived as a motive that drives behavior. It also involves an emotional component, a responsiveness *to*, an investment *in*, and a concern *for* another (Noddings, 1984). Although different from culture to culture, care almost always involves providing for the social, economic, physical, and/or emotional needs of someone else (Kolb, 2003). In this way care extends beyond merely an affective response.

Part of the social worker's function is to help clients clarify an ethical code of values in order to better guide their actions. Decision-making processes often depend on the ability of the social worker to mobilize the client's own wants, needs, and decision-making abilities. To accomplish these objectives, the feminist relational school emphasizes the practitioner's role in fostering mutuality and maximizing client participation. The client, and *only* the client, has to want to effect positive change. Mobilizing motivation and determination is an important part of the role of a social worker, who truly believes in the inherent desire of the client to move toward health. Acting on this belief lies at the heart of the strengths perspective and a feminist relational approach to practice.

Mutual respect, which grows out of engagement in a healthy connection, is an important part of the relational approach. When the worker is truly open to his or her own feelings, he or she can more easily resonate with and understand the client. Even in relationships where there is an unequal distribution of power, such as that between parent and child, listening to the other's experience, learning about the other's different perspectives, asking questions, sharing feelings, or telling stories can help to equalize the playing field. Consequently, both parties increase their understanding of each other, resulting in the growth of mutual respect (Miller, 2002).

## Self-Determination

Immanuel Kant was one of the leading modern philosophers who asserted that it is a person's right to determine his or her destiny (Loewenberg & Dolgoff, 1992). Maximizing opportunities for clients to make decisions about their own lives is inherent in applying this principle to social work practice (Freedberg, 1989). However, self-determination is not an absolute right. Much of the time, this concept, when applied to practice, is trumped by the lack of alternatives in a modern, hierarchical society, one in which certain people are limited by opportunity and privilege, laws and norms.

According to the NASW *Code of Ethics* (1999), "Social workers respect and promote the right of clients to self-determination and assist clients in their effort to identify and clarify their goals" (p. 4). In many ways, the notion of self-determination has become a source of one of the most common and perplexing dilemmas for social workers in working with women (Abramson, 1985). Women's available choices have historically been limited as a result of their diminished social status, their sense of autonomy compromised because of the oppression rooted in the social structures of a patriarchal society. Sometimes, without realizing it, females internalize the expectation that they should suppress their own needs in order to accommodate to the needs of others. One of the tasks for the social worker then is to help the client get in touch with her own will so she can have a better chance to actualize herself.

Before a woman can be helped to determine her life course, she must be empowered to believe she has the right to choose. Sometimes the seeds of empowerment are planted in the worker–client relationship, which ultimately affects other aspects of the client's life. Power imbalances exist in many relationships of women from diverse groups in society, so women may require help to understand the impact these power inequities may have on their sense of self and their right to self-determination. Patricia Hill Collins (1990) notes that the feminist method of understanding and explaining experience rests on the concept "the personal is political." Similarly, the feminist-relational approach offers a way of analyzing life and politics and the interactions between them. Political analysis of personal experience, the female experience in particular, fits well with an ecological-systems perspective, which entails understanding how the individual and the social environment intersect. As women come to know themselves and discover the role played by the political in defining their reality, they may ultimately change their conceptions of what they think they need and of the goals they set out to achieve. For social workers, helping women to achieve a more conscious recognition of the different influences that guide their behaviors may ultimately lead more women to discover their own voices.

## A Feminist Ethic of Care

Social work is about care. Irene Stiver (1997) highlights the multiple meanings the act of caring can have, observing that the giving of care usually implies a dependent arrangement. Sometimes the expression of caring is seen as interfering with the neutrality required in the therapeutic process. This "interference" has often been labeled countertransference, which infers that the worker is projecting her own needs and feelings onto the client. However, if the worker adheres to this view and is too cautious, the authentic connection that ultimately proves so powerful is hindered. The client needs to feel cared about. Caring is not only therapeutic, but also serves as a critical dimension of one's ability to adapt to complex environments, to establish and sustain relationships, and to enhance one's support base. All of these abilities may support a stronger sense of self and more effective coping strategies.

Caring also involves limit setting so that the balance between giver and receiver is not tipped in one direction or the other, except of course in the therapeutic relationship, where the focus is on the needs of the client, or in a relationship where one member is more dependent on the other because of age or disability. Even here, both individuals must seek proper balance. Many clients are involved in relationships that lack reciprocity, but in which mutual expressions of caring and concern could enhance their quality.

The objective of implementing a feminist ethic is to instill in clients a commitment to care as an important way to enhance their relationships and develop a greater sense of self and integrity. The ability to engage in a relationship that is marked by mutual care highlights the unique qualities of female development and implies a certain amount of strength and autonomy. Thus, a treatment goal in a client–worker relationship based on the feminist-relational model might be to enable the client to engage in relationships in which reciprocal caring is an active component, or at least to begin to work toward such relationships.

The feminist ethic of care emphasizes a longing for connection as the motivational force that underpins the development of women who have been socialized into a set of care-giving roles. Because the early social environment differs for males and females, women are more inclined to define themselves in relation to other people than are men (Chodorow, 1994). Thus, the desire for females to "do good," to assume responsibility for others, and to execute appropriate judgment is embedded in their conception of self and morality.

Many women hold a vision of relationships that gives rise to an ethic of justice and care. They hope that everyone will be treated equally, that everyone will be included, and that no one will be left alone. What gives this vision a feminist cast is its emphasis on the investment of feeling in the other person and the importance of mutuality. In other words, this ethic is rooted in relatedness, receptivity, and responsibility (Noddings, 1984).

When clients are in conflict over making decisions that affect their own lives and the lives of others, moral dilemmas are often expressed in terms of how to accommodate the client's personal needs and the needs of others without sacrificing the relationship entirely. The implication for social work practice is that interventions must be targeted toward working through that conflict with minimal damage.

Many times women who assume the role of caregiver do so because they believe they are following a normative role prescription. Conforming to the feminine ethic of care, the "morally mature" person understands and can negotiate the balance between caring for the self and caring for others (Freedberg, 1993). When a female client experiences conflict between competing responsibilities, the social worker needs to help her accept the idea that caring for herself is not selfish—that she can continue to care for others while continuing to care for herself at the same time.

Feminist scholarship has moved the field forward by providing a conceptual framework through which to analyze the role of the professional social worker in applying the feminist ethic of care. The central thesis of Carol Gilligan's landmark book, *In a Different Voice* (1982), is that a longing for connection is an important motivational force that underlies the moral development of women and results in the desire to care for others. Other forces impinging on women's prescription to care include how girls and women are socialized in a society that has largely bifurcated male and female expectations in relation to the commitment to care. Girls and women have been taught to define their sense of self and self-worth in relation to their nurturing and caretaking roles; boys and men have been taught to define their sense of self and self-worth in relation to their roles as providers and protectors. Of course, the feminine ethic of care can be learned by males as well.

The problem of reciprocity between the social worker (the one caring) and the client (the one cared for) is often one of balance, as it is in all relationships. What does each party contribute to the relationship and how does each meet the other on moral grounds? If the balance between worker and client is tipped too far to one side, the client may feel resentful, annoyed, overwhelmed, or taken advantage of. When this occurs, the relationship is strained and the client's functioning may then be compromised.

Gilligan (1982) found that women moved in and out of three moral frames of reference:

- Level I: overemphasis on an interest in themselves;
- Level II: overemphasis on an interest in others; and
- Level III: a balance between a healthy interest in themselves and a healthy interest in others.

Most women, consciously or not, have incorporated a commitment to care into their identities. Since society polarizes male and female roles, the feminist social worker must provide the opportunity for clients to experience a sense of connection, continuity, and belonging that allows them to create a socially responsible image of themselves. Awareness of the different socialization processes between women and men is important if we are to extend the notion of caring from the self to the family, to the social service agency, to the small group, to the organization, and to the community at large.

My focus on connection and disconnection speaks to the core of the human condition. Compassionate, care-centered practice focuses attention on maintaining a careful balance on the individual client and on salient social, political, and environmental factors that influence both clients' problems and society's responses, all with a sense of moral responsibility to the community at large (Hiersteiner et al. 1999). This position is consistent with the legacy of social work and the leaders who shaped our profession. In the 1930s and 1940s, Bertha Capen Reynolds (1963) and other social workers in the rank-and-file committed themselves to the union movement, not only to better wages and working conditions, but as an important vehicle to connect workers to each other and to the services they used.

However, today the principle of caring and compassion in social work too often lacks the context of a community of shared values. A model of mutuality and interdependence is a vision that the profession must continue to strive for, not only as a philosophy, but in order to invigorate our rich legacy of caring and responsibility for others, one that is vitally important, now more than ever.

# References

Abramson, M. (1985). The autonomy–paternalism dilemma in social work practice. *Social Casework*, 66(7), 387–393.

Agnew, E.N. (2004). *From charity to social reform*. Urbana, IL: University of Chicago Press.

Applegate, J.S. (1993). Winnicott and clinical social work: A facilitating partnership. *Child and Adolescent Social Work Journal*, 10(1), 3–19.

Astin, H.S. (1967). Assessment of empathic ability by means of a situational test. *Journal of Counseling Psychology*, 14(1), 57–60.

Basch, M.F. (1988). *Understanding psychotherapy*. New York: Basic Books.

Beebe, B. & Lachmann, F.M. (2002). *Infant research and adult treatment*. Hillsdale, NJ: Analytic Press.

Belenky, M.F., Clinchy, B.M., Goldberger, N.R. & Tarule, J.M. (1986). *Women's ways of knowing*. New York: Basic Books.

Benjamin, J. (1988). *Bonds of love*. New York: Pantheon.

Benjamin, J. (1995). *Like subjects, love objects: essays on recognition and sexual difference*. New Haven, CT: Yale University Press.

Benjamin, J. (1998). *Shadow of the other: Intersubjectivity and gender in psycho-analysis*. New York: Routledge.

Berger, D.M. (1987). *Clinical empathy*. Northvale, NJ: Jason Aronson.

Berzoff, J. (1989). From separation to connection: Shifts in understanding women's development. *Affilia: Journal of Women & Social Work*, 4(1), 45–58.

Berzoff, R., Melano Flanagan, L., & Hertz, P. (2004). Inside Out and Outside In. In *Psychodynamic clinical theory and practice in contemporary multicultural contexts*. A Jason Aronson Book, Oxford, UK: Rowman & Littlefield.

Biestek, F.P. (1957). *The casework relationship*. Chicago: Loyola University Press.

Bohart, A.C. & Greenberg, L.S. (Eds.) (1997). *Empathy reconsidered: New directions in psychotherapy*. Washington, DC: American Psychological Association.

Bowlby, J. (1969). *Attachment and loss*, Vol. I. New York: Basic Books.

Boyle, S.W., Hull, G.H., Mather, J.H., Smith, L.L., & Farley, W.O. (2006). *Direct practice in social work*. Boston: Allyn & Bacon.

Brazelton, T.B., Koslowski, B., & Main, M. (1974). *The origins of reciprocity: the early mother–infant interaction*. Hoboken, NJ: Wiley & Sons.

Casius, C. (Ed.) (1950). *A comparison of diagnostic and functional casework concepts*. New York: Family Service Association of America.

Chodorow, N. (1978). *The reproduction of mothering*. Berkeley, CA: University of California Press.

Chodorow, N.J. (1994). *Femininity, masculinities, sexualities*. Lexington, KY: Kentucky University Press.

Collins, B.G. (1986). Defining feminist social work. *Social Work*, *31*(3), 214–221.

Collins, P.H. (1990). *Black feminist thought: knowledge, consciousness, and the politics of empowerment*. New York: Routledge.

Compton, B.R., Galaway, B., & Cournoyer, B.R. (2005). *Social work processes*, 7th Edition. Belmont, CA: Brooks/Cole.

Cooper, M.G. & Lesser, J.G. (2002). *Clinical social work practice*. Boston: Allyn & Bacon.

Dewane, C.J. (2006). Use of self: A primer revisited. *Clinical Social Work Journal*, *34*(4), 543–558.

Dinnerstein, D. (1997) *The mermaid and the minotaur*. New York: Harper Books.

Dyche, L. & Zayas, L.H. (2001). Cross-cultural empathy and training the contemporary psychotherapist. *Clinical Social Work Journal*, *29*(3), 245–258.

Edwards, R.L. (Ed.) (1995). *Encyclopedia of social work*. Vol. 3, 19th Edition. Washington, DC: National Association of Social Workers.

Ehrenreich, J. (1985). *The altruist imagination*. Ithaca, NY: Cornell University Press.

Eisenberg, N. & Strayer, J. (1987). Critical issues in the study of empathy. In N. Eisenberg & J. Strayer (Eds.), *Empathy and development* (pp. 3–16). Cambridge, UK: Cambridge University Press.

Erikson, E.H. (1950). *Childhood and society*. New York: Norton.

Erikson, E.H. (1968). *Identity: youth and crisis*. London: Faber & Faber.

Family Service Society of America. (1958). *Method and process in social casework*. Report of a staff committee of the Community Service Society of New York. New York.

Fonagy, P. (2001). *Attachment theory and psychoanalysis*. New York: Other Press.

Fox, R. (2001). *Elements of the helping process*. Binghamton, NY: Haworth Press.

Freedberg, S. (1984). Bertha Capen Reynolds: A woman out of step with her times. Unpublished doctoral dissertation, Columbia University.

Freedberg, S. (1989). Self-determination: Historical perspectives and effects on current practice. *Social Work*, *34*(1), 33–38.

Freedberg, S. (1993). The feminine ethic of care and the professionalization of social work. *Social Work*, *38*(5), 535–540.

Freud, S. (1923/1961). The ego and the id. In J. Strachey (Ed. and Trans.), *The standard edition of the complete psychological works of Sigmund Freud*, Vol. 20. London: Hogarth Press.

Garrett, A. (1958). The worker–client relationship. In H.J. Parad (Ed.), *Ego psychology and dynamic casework* (p. 53). New York: Family Service Association of America.

Gaylin, W. (1978). The limits of benevolence. In W. Gaylin, I.M. Glaser, & D. Rothman (Eds.), *Doing good* (pp. 1–39). New York: Pantheon.

Genero, N.P., Miller, J.B., Surrey, J., & Baldwin, L.M. (1992). Measuring perceived mutuality in close relationships: Validation of the mutual psychological development questionnaire. *Journal of Family Psychology*, *6*(1), 36–48.

Germain, C.B. (1970). Casework and science: A scientific encounter. In R.W. Roberts & R.H. Nee (Eds.), *Theories of social casework* (pp. 3–33). Chicago: University of Chicago Press.

Germain, C.B. (1991). *Human behavior in the social environment: An ecological view*. New York: Columbia University Press.

Germain, C.B. & Gitterman, A. (1996). *The life model of social work practice*, 2nd edition. New York: Columbia University Press.

Gilligan, C. (1982). *In a different voice: Psychological theory and women's development*. Cambridge, MA: Harvard University Press.

Goldstein, E. (1984). *Ego psychology and social work practice*. New York: Free Press.

Greenberg, J.R. & Mitchell, S.A. (1983). *Object relations in psychoanalytic theory*. Cambridge, MA: Harvard University Press.

Griffin, D.W. & Bartholomew, K. (1994). The metaphysics of measurement: The case of adult attachment. In K. Bartholomew & D. Perlman (Eds.), *Advances in personal relationships, Vol. 5: Attachment processes in adulthood* (pp. 17–52). London: Jessica Kingsley Publishers.

Guntrip, H.J.S. (1971). *Psychoanalytic theory, therapy, and the self*. New York: Basic Books.

Hamilton, G. (1951). *Theory and practice of social casework*. New York: Columbia University Press.

Hepworth, D.H., Rooney, R.H., Rooney, G.D., Strom-Gottfried, K., & Larsen, J. (2006). *Direct social work practice, theory, and skills*. Belmont, CA: Thomson.

Hiersteiner, C. & Peterson, K.J. (1999). "Crafting a usable past": The care-centered practice narrative in social work. *Affilia, 14*(2), 144–161.

Hill, O. (1875). *Homes of the London poor*. New York: Macmillan.

Hochschild, A.R. & Machung, A. (2003). *The second shift*. New York: Penguin Books.

Hoffman, M. (1997). Sex differences in empathy and related behaviors. *Psychological Bulletin, 84*(4), 712–722.

Hollis, F. (1964/1981). *Casework: A psychological therapy*. New York: Random House.

Jordan, J.V. (1983). Empathy in the mother–daughter relationship. In J.V. Jordan, J.L. Surrey, & A. Kaplan (Eds.), *Women and empathy* (Working Paper Series, Work in Progress, No. 82, pp. 2–5). Wellesley, MA: Stone Center.

Jordan, J.V. (1984). *Empathy and self-boundaries* (Working Paper Series, Work in Progress, No. 16). Wellesley, MA: Stone Center Working Paper Series.

Jordan, J.V. (1986). The meaning of mutuality (Working Paper Series, Work in Progress, No. 23). Wellesley, MA: Stone Center Working Paper Series.

Jordan, J.V. (1989). *Relational development: Therapeutic implications of empathy and shame* (Working Paper Series, Work in Progress, No. 39). Wellesley, MA: Stone Center.

Jordan, J.V. (1991a). Empathy and self-boundaries. In J.V. Jordan, A.G. Kaplan, J.B. Miller, I.P. Stiver, & J.L. Surrey (Eds.), *Women's growth in connection* (pp. 67–80). New York: Guilford Press.

Jordan, J.V. (1991b). Empathy, mutuality and therapeutic change: Clinical implications of a relational model. In J.V. Jordan, A.G. Kaplan, J.B. Miller, I.P. Stiver, & J.L. Surrey (Eds.), *Women's growth in connection* (pp. 283–290). New York: Guilford Press.

Jordan, J.V. (1991c). The meaning of mutuality. In J.V. Jordan, A.G. Kaplan, J.B. Miller, I.P. Stiver, & J.L. Surrey (Eds.), *Women's growth in connection* (pp. 81–96). New York: Guilford Press.

Jordan, J.V. (1991d). *The movement of mutuality and power* (Working Paper Series, Working in Progress, No. 53). Wellesley, MA: The Stone Center.

Jordan, J.V. (1994). *A relational perspective on self-esteem* (Working Paper Series, Working Paper No. 70). Wellesley, MA: The Stone Center.

Jordan, J.V. (1997a). A relational perspective for understanding women's development. In J.V. Jordan (Ed.), *Women's growth in diversity: More writings from the Stone Center* (pp. 9–24). New York: Guilford Press.

Jordan, J.V. (1997b). The relational model as a source of empowerment for women. In M.R. Walsh (Ed.), *Women, men, and gender: Ongoing debates* (pp. 373–382). New Haven, CT: Yale University Press.

Jordan, J.V. (2004). Toward competence and connection. In J.V. Jordan, M. Walker, & L.M. Hartling (Eds.), *The complexity of connection: Writings from the Stone Center's Jean Baker Miller Training Institute* (pp. 11–28). New York: Guilford Press.

Jordan, J.V. & Dooley, C. (2000). *Relational practice in action: A group manual.* (Jean Baker Miller Training Institute, Project Report, No. 6). Wellesley, MA: Stone Center.

Jordan, J.V., Kaplan, A.G., Miller, J.B., Stiver, I.P., & Surrey, J.L. (1991). *Women's growth in connection: Writings from the Stone Center.* New York: Guilford Press.

Jordan, J.V., Surrey, J.L., & Kaplan, A.G. (1991). Women and empathy: Implications for psychological development and psychotherapy. In J.V. Jordan, A.G. Kaplan, J.B. Miller, I.P. Stiver, & J.L. Surrey (Eds.), *Women's growth in connection* (pp. 27–50). New York: Guilford Press.

Jordan, J.V., Walker, M., & Hartling, L.M. (Eds.) (2004). *The complexity of connection: Writings from the Stone Center's Jean Baker Miller Training Institute.* New York: Guilford Press.

Kaplan, A.G. (1988). *Dichotomous thought and relational processes in therapy* (Working Paper Series, Work in Progress, No. 35). Wellesley, MA: Stone Center.

Kaplan, A.G. (1991). The "self-in-relation": Implications for depression in women. In J.V. Jordan, A.G. Kaplan, J.B. Miller, I.P. Stiver, & J.L. Surrey (Eds.), *Women's growth in connection* (pp. 206–222). New York: Guilford Press.

Kaplan, A.G., Klein, R., & Gleason, N. (1985). *Women's self development in late adolescence* (Working Paper Series, Work in Progress, No. 17). Wellesley, MA: Stone Center.

Keefe, T. (1976). The development of empathic skill: A study. *Journal of Education for Social Work, 15*(2), 30–38.

Kernberg, O.F. (1976). *Object relations theory and clinical psychoanalysis.* Northvale, NJ: Jason Aronson.

Kimmel, M. (Ed.) (2004). *The gendered society.* New York: Oxford University Press.

Kirst-Ashman, K. & Hull, G. (1995). *Understanding generalist practice.* Chicago: Nelson-Hall Publishers.

Kohlberg, L. (1981). *Essays on moral development, Vol. I: The philosophy of moral development.* New York: Harper & Row.

Kohut, H. (1977). *The restoration of the self.* New York: International Universities Press.

Kolb, P. (2003). *Caring for our elders.* New York: Columbia University Press.

Kuhn, T.S. (1970). *The structure of scientific revolutions.* Chicago: University of Chicago Press.

Lacan, J. (1985). *Feminine sexuality.* New York: W.W. Norton.

Laing, B., Taylor, C., Williams, L.M., Tracy, A., Jordan, J.V., & Miller, J.B. (1998).

*The relational health indices: An exploratory study*. Wellesley, MA: Wellesley Centers for Women.

Levine, E.R. (2002). Glossary. In A.R. Roberts & G.J. Greene (Eds.), *Social work desk reference* (pp. 829–849). New York: Oxford University Press.

Levinson, D.J. (1978). *The seasons of a man's life*. New York: Ballentine Books.

Loewenberg, F.M. & Dolgoff, R. (1992). *Ethical decisions for social work practice*. Itasca, IL: F.E. Peacock Publishers.

Lubove, R. (1969). *Professional altruist: The emergence of social work as a career 1880–1930*. New York: Atheneum.

Lucas, Keith-A. (1976). *Giving and taking help*. St. Davids, PA: North American Association of Christians in Social Work.

Mahler, M.S., Pine, F., & Bergman, A. (1975). *The psychological birth of the human infant: Symbiosis and individuation*. New York: Basic Books.

Marsh, J.C. (2005). Social work: Help starts here. *Social Work, 50*(3), 195–196.

Meyer, C.H. (1993). *Assessment in social work practice*. New York: Columbia University Press.

Miller, J.B. (1976). *Toward a new psychology of women*. Boston: Beacon Press.

Miller, J.B. (1991a). The construction of anger in women and men. In J.V. Jordan, A.G. Kaplan, J.B. Miller, I.P. Stiver, & J.L. Surrey (Eds.), *Women's growth in connection* (pp. 181–196). New York: Guilford Press.

Miller, J.B. (1991b). The development of women's sense of self. In J.V. Jordan, A.G. Kaplan, J.B. Miller, I.P. Stiver, & J.L. Surrey (Eds.), *Women's growth in connection* (pp. 11–26). New York: Guilford Press.

Miller, J.B. (1991c). Women and power. In J.V. Jordan, A.G. Kaplan, J.B. Miller, I.P. Stiver, & J.L. Surrey (Eds.), *Women's growth in connection* (pp. 197–205). New York: Guilford Press.

Miller, J.B. (2002). *How change happens: Controlling images, mutuality, and power* (Working Paper Series, Work in Progress, No. 96). Wellesley, MA: Stone Center.

Miller, J.B., Jordan, J.V., Kaplan, A.G., Stiver, I.P., & Surrey, J.L. (1997). Some misconceptions and reconceptions of a relational approach. In J.V. Jordan (Ed.), *Women's growth in diversity: More writings from the Stone Center* (pp. 25–49). New York: Guilford Press.

Miller, J.B., Jordan, J.V., Stiver, I.P., Walker, M., Surrey, J.L., & Eldridge, N.S. (1999). *Therapists' authenticity* (Working Paper Series, Work in Progress, No, 82). Wellesley, MA: Stone Center.

Miller, J.B. & Stiver, I.P. (1991). *A relational reframing of therapy*. (Working Paper Series, Work in Progress, No. 52). Wellesley, MA: Stone Center.

Miller, J.B. & Stiver, I.P. (1995). *Relational images and their meaning in psychotherapy* (Working Paper Series, Work in Progress, No. 74). Wellesley, MA: Stone Center.

Miller, J.B. & Stiver, I.P. (1997). *The healing connection: How women form relationships in therapy and in life*. Boston: Beacon Press.

Minahan, A. (Ed.) (1986). *Encyclopedia of social work*, 18th Edition. Washington, DC: National Association of Social Workers.

Mitchell, S.A. (1988). *Relational concepts in psychoanalysis: An integration*. Cambridge, MA: Harvard University Press.

Mitchell, S.A. & Black, M.J. (1995). *Freud and beyond*. New York: Basic Books.

National Association of Social Workers (1999). *Code of ethics*. Washington, DC: Author.

Noddings, N. (1984). *Caring: A feminine approach to ethics and moral education.* Berkeley, CA: University of California Press.

Perlman, H.H. (1957). *Casework: A problem-solving process.* Chicago: University of Chicago Press.

Perlman, H.H. (1979). *Relationship: The heart of helping people.* Chicago: University of Chicago Press.

Phillips, N.K. & Straussner, L.A.S. (2002). *Urban social work.* Boston: Allyn & Bacon.

Pinderhughes, E. (1979). Teaching empathy in cross-cultural social work. *Social Work, 24*(4), 312–316.

Pumphrey, R.E. & Pumphrey, M.W. (1961). *The heritage of American social work.* New York: Columbia University Press.

Raines, J.C. (1990). Empathy in clinical social work. *Clinical Social Work Journal, 18*(1), 57–72.

Raines, J.C. (1996). Self-disclosure in clinical social work. *Clinical Social Work Journal, 24*(4), 357–375.

Reiter, L. (1995). The client's affective impact on the therapist: Implications for therapist responsiveness. *Clinical Social Work Journal, 23*(1), 21–35.

Reynolds, B.C. (1951). *Social work and social living.* Silver Spring, MD: National Association of Social Workers.

Reynolds, B.C. (1963). *An uncharted journey.* New York: Citadel Press.

Rhodes, M.L. (1985). Gilligan's theory of moral development as applied to social work. *Social Work, 30*(2), 101–106.

Richmond, M.E. (1899). *Friendly visiting among the poor: A handbook for charity workers.* New York: Charity Organization Society of New York.

Richmond, M.E. (1917). *Social diagnosis.* New York: Russell Sage.

Richmond, M.E. (1922). *What is social casework? An introductory description.* New York: Russell Sage Foundation.

Robinson, V.P. (1930). *A changing psychology in social casework.* Chapel Hill, NC: University of North Carolina Press.

Rogers, C. (1951). *Client-centered therapy.* New York: Houghton Mifflin.

Rowe, C.E. & Mac Isaac, D.S. (1991). *Empathic attunement: The technique of psychoanalytic self psychology.* Northvale, NJ: Jason Aronson.

Rutter, M. (1990). Psychosocial resilience and protective mechanisms. In J. Rolf, A.S. Masten, D. Cicchetti, K.H. Nuechterlein, & S. Weintraub (Eds.), *Risk and protective factors in the development of psychopathology* (pp. 181–214). New York: Cambridge University Press.

Sands, R.G. & Nuccio, K. (1992). Post-modern feminist theory and social work. *Social Work, 37*(6), 489–494.

Shulman, L. (2006) *The skills of helping individuals, families, groups, and communities.* Belmont, CA: Thomson.

Smalley, R. (1970). The functional approach to casework. In R.W. Roberts & R.H. Nee (Eds.), *Theories of Social Casework* (pp. 77–129). Chicago: University of Chicago Press.

Smalley, R. & and Bloom, T. (1977). Social casework: The functional approach. In J.B. Turner (Ed.) *Encyclopedia of social work*, 17th Edition, pp. 1280–1290.

Smith, K.F., Goodman, L., & Glenn, C. (2006). The full-frame approach: A new response to marginalized women left behind by specialized services. *American Journal of Orthopsychiatry, 76*(4), 489–502.

Smith, R.F. (1977). Settlements and neighborhood centers. In *Encyclopedia of social work*. 19th Edition (Vol. 3, pp. 2129–2135) Washington, DC: National Association of Social Workers.

Spencer, R. (2000). *A comparison of relational psychologies* (Working Paper Series, Project Report, No. 5). Wellesley, MA: Wellesley Centers for Women.

St. Clair, M. (2004). *Object relations and self psychology: An introduction*. Belmont, CA: Thomson/Brooks/Cole.

Stern, D.N. (1985). *The interpersonal world of the infant: A view from psycho-analysis and development psychology*. New York: Basic Books.

Stiver, I.P. (1991). The meanings of "dependency" in female-male relationships. In J.V. Jordan, A.G. Kaplan, J.B. Miller, I.P. Stiver, & J.L. Surrey (Eds.), *Women's growth in connection* (pp. 143–161). New York: Guilford Press.

Stiver, I.P. (1997). A relational approach to therapeutic impasses. In J.V. Jordan (Ed.), *Women's growth in diversity: More writings from the Stone Center* (pp. 288–310). New York: Guilford Press.

Stiver, I.P. & Miller, J.B. (1988). *From depression to sadness in women's psycho-therapy* (Working Paper Series, Work in Progress, No. 36). Wellesely, MA: Stone Center.

Stiver, I.P. & Miller, J.B. (1997). From depression to sadness in women's psycho-therapy. In J.V. Jordan (ed.), *Women's growth in diversity: More writings from the Stone Center* (pp. 217–238). New York: Guilford Press.

Stolorow, R.D., Atwood, G.E., & Brandchaft, B. (Eds.) (1994). *The intersubjective perspective*. Northvale, NJ: Jason Aronson.

Sullivan, H.S. (1940). *Conceptions of modern psychology*. New York: William Allison White Psychiatric Foundation.

Surrey, J.L. (1987). *Relationships and empowerment* (Working Paper Series, Work in Progress, No. 30). Wellesley, MA: Stone Center.

Surrey, J.L. (1991). The "self-in-relation": A theory of women's development. In J.V. Jordan, A.G. Kaplan, J.B. Miller, I.P. Stiver, & J.L. Surrey (Eds.), *Women's growth in connection* (pp. 51–66). New York: Guilford Press.

Surrey, J.L. (1997). What do you mean by mutuality? In J.V. Jordan (ed.), *Women's growth in diversity: More writings from the Stone Center* (pp. 42–49). New York: Guilford Press.

Surrey, J.L., Kaplan, A., & Jordan, J.V. (1990). *Empathy revisited* (Working Paper Series, Work in Progress, No. 40). Wellesley, MA: Stone Center.

Tronick, E.Z. & Weinberg, M.K. (1997). Depressed mothers and infants: Failure to form dyadic states of consciousness. In L. Murray & P.J. Cooper (Eds.), *Postpartum depression and child development* (pp. 54–81). New York: Guilford Press.

Tropp, E. (1977). Social group work: The development approach. In J.B. Turner (ed.), *Encyclopedia of social work*, Vol. 11, 17th Edition (pp. 1321–1327). Washington, DC: National Association of Social Workers.

Truax, C.B. & Mitchell, K.M. (1971). Research on certain therapist interpersonal skills in relation to process and outcome. In A.E. Bergin & S.L. Garfield (Eds.), *Handbook of psychotherapy and behavior change* (pp. 299–344). New York: John Wiley & Sons.

Turner, C.W. (1997). Clinical applications of the Stone Center theoretical approach to minority women. In J.V. Jordan (ed.), *Women's growth in diversity: More writings from the Stone Center* (pp. 74–90). New York: Guilford Press.

Walker, M. (2004). How relationships heal. In M. Walker & W.B. Rosen (Eds.), *How connections heal: Stories from relational–cultural therapy* (pp. 3–22). New York: Guilford Press.

Wenocur, S. & Reisch, M. (1989). *From charity to enterprise: The development of American social work in a market economy.* Urbana, IL: University of Illinois Press.

Werner, E.E. (1989). High-risk children in young adulthood: a longitudinal study from birth to 32 years. *American Journal of Orthopsychiatry, 59*(1), 72–81.

White, R. (1963). *Ego and reality in psychoanalytic theory.* New York: International Universities Press.

Winnicott, D.W. (1965). *The maturational processes and the facilitating environment.* New York: International Universities Press.

Wishnie, H.A. (2005). *Working in the counter-transference: Necessary entanglements.* London, UK: Rowman & Littlefield.

Woods, M.E. & Hollis, F. (1999). *Casework: A psychosocial therapy* (5th Edition). New York: McGraw-Hill.

# Index